M000314699

Praise for **PRAYFIT**

In boxing, there is no room for error. You have to not only be physically prepared but also spiritually strong. Being a big believer in Jesus Christ, *PrayFit* gets me on track to start my day in the right direction.

Robert "The Ghost" Guerrero
Three-Time World Boxing Champion

This exciting devotional, *PrayFit*, will enable you to live out the Scripture that says, "Love the Lord your God with all your heart and with all your soul and with all your mind and with all your strength!" (Mark 12:30).

Josh Hamilton
Major League Baseball All-Star Outfielder
MVP of the 2010 American League Championship Series

Jimmy Peña is one of the most knowledgeable fitness writers I know. He's one of our nation's leading fitness resources. Respect.

LL Cool J
Actor/Entertainer

In *PrayFit*, Jimmy Peña brings his expertise as a physical trainer and his passion for walking closer to the Lord together in a powerful way. Each of the readings in this book will encourage you physically and help you grow closer to the Lord. Working in tandem with the Holy Spirit, you will change your life on every level—physical, mental, emotional and spiritual.

Carole Lewis
National Director, First Place 4 Health
Author, *Give God a Year* and *Hope 4 You*

Not only is Jimmy Peña one of my best friends, but whenever I want to get dialed-in for a role or photo shoot, he's also my only call. And I love starting my day at www.PrayFit.com, building spiritual and physical muscle. A one-of-a-kind concept from the best in the business.

Mario Lopez
Host, *EXTRA*

PrayFit is packed with a lot of helpful and interesting information. It provides a systematic plan for building your spiritual and physical health. Read and apply it for a better life.

Steve Reynolds
Pastor, Capital Baptist Church, Annandale, Virginia
Author, *Bod4God: Four Keys to Weight Loss*

Clinical Exercise Physiologist and *New York Times* Bestselling Author

JIMMY PEÑA

WITH **JIMMY PAGE, MS** AND **JIM STOPPANI, PHD**

✝PRAYFIT™

YOUR GUIDE TO A HEALTHY BODY AND A STRONGER FAITH IN 28 DAYS

INCLUDES DEVOTIONS, EXERCISES AND MEAL PLANS

Regal

From Gospel Light
Ventura, California, U.S.A.

Published by Regal
From Gospel Light
Ventura, California, U.S.A.
www.regalbooks.com
Printed in the U.S.A.

Caution: The information contained in this book is intended solely for information and
educational purposes. It is assumed that the reader will consult a medical or health
professional before beginning this or any other weight-loss or physical fitness program.

Library of Congress Cataloging-in-Publication Data
Peña, Jimmy.
Prayfit : your guide to a healthy body and a stronger faith in 28 days /
Jimmy Peña with Jimmy Page and Jim Stoppani.
p. cm.
ISBN 978-0-8307-5651-3 (hardcover)
1. Christian men—Religious life. 2. Christian men—Health and hygiene.
I. Page, Jimmy. II. Stoppani, James, 1968- III. Title.
IV. Title: Your guide to a healthy body and a stronger faith in 28 days.
BV4528.2.P45 2010
248.4—dc22
2010029913

3 4 5 6 7 8 9 10 11 12 13 / 20 19 18 17 16 15 14 13 12 11

To Henry and Sandie Powell

If God made better, sweeter people, I've never met them.
Thank you for your love for the Lord and your lifetime of evangelism.
I gladly dedicate this book to you.
Because of your "profession of faith," I have mine.

Contents

Month One: Decision Day
28 Days to Fitness

Month One: Dig a Little Deeper
28 Bonus Days to Help Keep You on Track

Keep Praying and Stay Fit!

A great man named Bill Parcells once told me, "There's a big difference between routine and commitment. Most people do the same routine over and over, but few people commit to the next level."

Whether you're a beginner or a veteran in your pursuit of a stronger body, or of a stronger relationship with God, *PrayFit* will encourage you to ascend beyond the normal routine and inspire you to commit to the next level.

When we consider our health, we tend to consider only the physical aspects. *Am I eating the right foods? Am I exercising enough?* But the body is only one facet of our being. What about our spiritual health? We operate as a whole, with all parts connected: body, mind and spirit. Each part is essential to and affected by the others. If a spot on an apple is left to rot, does it not eventually spoil the whole fruit? We must focus on developing ourselves in totality rather than compartmentally. As we are mindful of how we eat and exercise, we must also be mindful of how we think and what we believe.

Often, we fail to realize that when we open ourselves up physically, our minds are prepared to follow. Think about it—after a workout, it's fair to say that we get an overall sense of wellbeing and accomplishment. We just feel good! In terms of spirituality, it makes perfect sense that as we open ourselves up physically and connect to the vessel that God has given us (our body), we naturally begin to feel a connection to all of God's work. It's as though the connection with God becomes more tangible.

During my career in the NFL, I've seen some of the world's most physically gifted athletes lose their careers due to a lack of strong moral character. I've also seen some of the most devout spiritual leaders jeopardize themselves because they were physically unfit. *PrayFit* focuses on the importance of a balanced life—a life committed to both physical and spiritual nourishment, and one that flourishes when faith and fitness intersect.

Keep praying and stay fit!

Curtis Martin

Curtis Martin was a five-time NFL Pro Bowl selection during his 11-year career with the New England Patriots and New York Jets, and captured league Offensive Rookie of the Year honors in 1995.

Why PRAYFIT?

I know beyond a shadow of a doubt that this life is not about the body (and aren't we glad for that?). As C. S Lewis said, "You don't have a soul. You are a soul. You have a body." I'm so thankful that someday I'll turn this body in for a brand-new one. But in the short term—during my time in this temporary home—I've been called to a lifetime commitment of greater health and wellness. Not just so I can feel great and have more energy, which are all benefits from exercise, but even more because I believe we've been called to a higher standard in the area of physical health.

My dad used to tell me that how I cared for the truck he gave me was an indication of how much I appreciated the gift. Keeping it clean and maintained was a way to show him love in return. And if I took care of it, I could extend its life and improve its efficiency. I think in some way the same can be said about how God has gifted us with our bodies. How well we take care of them can, in some ways, be a means to show our love in return. Our efforts to maintain healthy habits are a way of saying, "Thank You, God, for life, for ability, for opportunity and for the air in my lungs, because it's You who breathed it there in the first place. I'm going to live my life to the fullest, in Jesus' name."

And so we can say with absolute certainty that *PrayFit* is not about perfection but about obedience and discipline. The goal of *PrayFit* is not a better pair of biceps, but a pursuit of the healthiest possible version of the body He gave us so that we can better fulfill our purpose, whatever the calling might be.

Fitness and faith is the intersection at which I've been called to serve for the rest of my life. And until Jesus comes back or calls me home, I'm going to pursue physical and spiritual excellence on a daily basis. And someday, when I exchange this body for one that's new, I hope He's proud of the inner and outer man I gave Him in return.

Best Efforts

At its core, *PrayFit* is about giving your daily best effort in two areas that are vital to your wellbeing: faith and fitness.

As you go through the book, each day will begin with a brief devotional written by either me or my trusted friend and associate, Jimmy Page, of Fellowship of Christian Athletes (FCA). Page serves as Vice President of Field Ministry and National Director of Wellness for Fellowship of Christian Athletes (FCA). For nearly 20 years, he has been a leader in the medical fitness industry, operating wellness facilities affiliated with Sinai Hospital and Johns Hopkins. He currently hosts a daily radio segment and podcast called "Fit Life Today," offering a blend of spiritual and physical health principles that promote abundant life. In 2010, Page published *Wisdom Walks: 40 Life-Changing Principles to Live and Give. Wisdom Walks* is a field manual for mentoring the next generation and can be found at www.wisdomwalks.org.

As an author, speaker, ordained minister and trainer, Page's passion is to challenge people to transform their life and walk with Jesus, and we are blessed to have him as a co-author on Prayfit's first publication.

You'll follow—or precede—each devotional with a workout that you can do in the comfort of your living room with little to no equipment. I've put this program together in a way that will challenge you in ways you didn't think possible, mainly through your own body weight. Couple this progressive fitness program with daily tips that you can file away for a healthier overall lifestyle and you're well on your way to abundant living.

But as you may already know, nutrition can make or break your progress with your fitness goals. That's why we tasked one of the country's top nutrition minds to map out a meal plan anyone can follow—not just for a few weeks, but also in perpetuity. Dr. Jim Stoppani, the senior science editor for *Muscle & Fitness, Muscle & Fitness Hers* and *Flex* magazines, knows that extreme dieting is not only dangerous and detrimental to your build, but that it is impossible to sustain. His expert nutritional advice will help you maximize the benefits of the fitness plan by simply reapportioning the foods you're probably already eating. His wealth of experience is a fantastic resource to the PrayFit team.

In addition to his magazine work, Dr. Stoppani is a science consultant for numerous companies. He has written hundreds of articles on exercise, diet and health and is author of the book *Encyclopedia of Muscle & Strength* (Human Kinetics, 2006); co-author of the chapter "Nutritional Needs of Strength/Power Athletes" in the textbook *Essentials of Sports Nutrition and Supplements* (Humana Press, 2008); co-author of the book *Stronger Arms & Upper Body* (Human Kinetics, 2008); co-author of the sequel to the *New York Times* bestseller, *LL Cool J's Platinum Workout* (Rodale, 2007); LL Cool J's *Platinum Nutrition* (Rodale, 2009); and contributor to Mario Lopez's *Knockout Fitness* (Rodale, 2008). He is also the personal nutrition and health consultant for numerous celebrity clients, such as Dr. Dre, LL Cool J and Mario Lopez. He has appeared on the NBC television show *Extra* as an *Extra* LifeChanger and as a science expert for Spike television.

Crossing Paths

Reinforcing your relationship with the Lord and seeking abundant health shouldn't be mutually exclusive goals, since He calls us to give attention to both. The reason for that is simple—so that we may be fitter as we walk with Him through life. This charge is the backbone principle of *PrayFit*: daily quiet time with the Lord and a daily appointment with exercise. Each day is a chance to achieve balance, become as strong as we are studied, as fit as we are faithful and maintain personal accountability in a way that pleases Him. That's something that we should all strive for.

At PrayFit, we believe God gives us strength for today, offering no assurances about tomorrow. It makes sense then that we should capitalize on each day, powering through as bold, loving servants, constantly finding ways to nurture our mind, body and spirit. He wants us to remember that our faith is all about relationship. He wants us to walk with Him, not just for Him. Conversing with Him and living in His Word on a daily basis are like water for your soul—you need it to thrive, period. We believe that anything good in us comes from Christ, and apart from Him we can't do or be anything at all. Are you giving your best in the area of quiet study moments?

From a physical standpoint, physical inactivity isn't just detrimental to your wardrobe; each passing day of inactivity or nutritional indiscretion is a missed opportunity to live a longer, healthier, more fruitful life among friends and family. When a daily walk or a few bodyweight exercises are all that's standing between you and a stronger, leaner, more efficient body, you have to ask yourself: Are you giving your best effort with your body?

For that reason, we believe *PrayFit* offers the solution to the lack of daily prayer and exercise among believers. Because in a nation gone mad with super-sized meal deals, even the most devout believers tend to overindulge, as evidenced by America's collective and ever-widening waistline. We've also become smooth-kneed in the area of carving out time to read and study the Bible. I suppose you could say *PrayFit* is both preventive medicine and healing treatment for physical and spiritual heart disease.

PrayFit can help you give your best effort in both areas by providing the daily prescription for the inner and outer man or woman. For 28 days, you'll travel a path—along with fellow *PrayFit* participants and those who make up your personal support structure—toward greater spiritual awareness and confidence, and a physique that's better for the journey. (There 28 days of bonus *PrayFit* exercises after the first month to help keep you on track.)

So, won't you join us? We'll be at the intersection of fitness and faith, with you on our minds.

PrayFit:

Training Your Faith and Your Body

Training Your Faith

I often suggest to people that they pair up with a workout partner who is stronger and further along in his or her sport, in order to be stretched beyond their normal limits. For that reason, Jimmy Page, my friend, ordained minister and counselor, has laid the foundation of faith between the covers of *PrayFit*. His heart and love for the Lord, and his biblical insight, will be a reservoir for you, as they have been for me. Listen as he describes his perspective on the importance of daily quiet time with God, in his own words:

> For years, I thought I could grow spiritually and become a man of God by going to church on Sunday, getting in a quick, five-minute devotion in the morning and praying over my meals. I regularly compared where I was spiritually with others, and since I was also leading a Bible study and was involved in men's ministry at my church, I figured I was in better shape than most in my pursuit of God.
>
> But the reality was this—most of the time I was just playing around with my faith. I didn't spend enough time with God to actually grow or experience significant life change.
>
> What I was doing was the equivalent of a spiritual warm-up. I rarely, if ever, got to the training part! And I certainly didn't have

much of a plan. As a result, I had the appearance of godliness without much transformational experience. I had a great reputation, but my words lacked wisdom, my attitude lacked humility, my heart lacked compassion and my life lacked power. What I've found is that my experience is pretty common. In fact, there's a good chance that you've felt this way as well and may even be experiencing this right now.

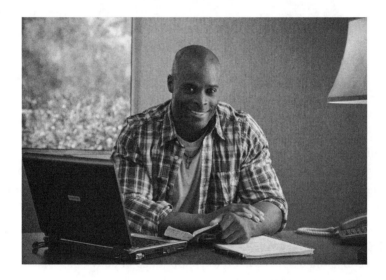

In 1 Timothy 4:7-8, Paul says, "Train yourself to be godly. For physical training is of some value, but godliness has value for all things, holding promise for both the present life and the life to come." In other words, physical training is good, but spiritual training is better. And I believe the two go hand in hand. Paul is making the case that if you want to grow spiritually, if you want to be changed on the inside, you will have to train.

For many of us, our spiritual life probably mirrors our physical. We make resolutions and have good intentions to get in shape. We get off to a good start with exercise and eating better, and we even start to feel so good that we wonder why we ever stopped the last time. We see results, and our friends even tell us that they see a difference. They even ask what we're doing because they want what we have—energy, enthusiasm, weight loss and strength. And then, almost inevitably, the chaos of life gets in the way and we get derailed. In order to get stronger in our relationship with God, it's going to take a sacrifice of time, effort and energy. Can you even imagine what life might look like if we put as much time and energy into "spiritual exercise" as we do the physical?

I have personally experienced the life-changing power of God's Word, and I know you will too. Join us as we do whatever it takes to reconnect with God, renew our mind and refresh our soul.

Thanks, brother. And so, with Page's help, we've created a spiritual training program that gives you what you need each day to grow closer to Jesus. With *PrayFit,* you will read the life-changing Word of God. You will be pushed to take a clear look at your life, to let God reveal areas that need change, and then to put these biblical principles into practice. You will have an opportunity to pray and record your thoughts and even memorize key verses that encourage your faith to grow.

On each page, you'll encounter these elements in clearly laid out sections:

1. **The Exercise**: A daily reading followed by a broader study designed to help you get more out of Scripture.

2. **Pastor's Point**: A question—or two, or three—designed to provoke thought on the day's reading and what it might tell you about God's will for your life. This section will also include additional verses that further illustrate the day's lesson.

3. **Walking with Him**: Consider this your spiritual exercise for the day. This faith-based directive will help you take steps toward a deeper relationship with the Lord.

4. **Journal Space**: Use this space to jot down your reaction to that day's reading, lay out goals or to note interesting points about the study that you'd like to revisit.

Training Your Body

PrayFit is all about daily decisions. In fact, the *PrayFit* philosophy that we've designed is built on the foundation of minute-by-minute, day-by-day decisions. The mere fact that you're reading the words on this page is a testament to your God-given, strive-to-be-better nature. Somewhere deep inside your gut you've made a decision: You're going to take back your health. And now that you're committing to make better food choices and spend a few minutes training the inner and outer man, you might be asking yourself, "Where do I start?" We understand.

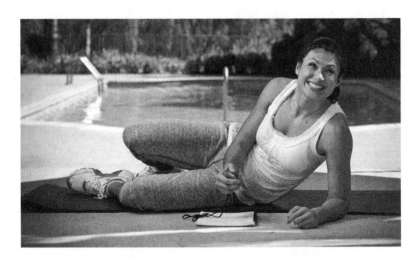

Step into the magazine aisle of your local bookstore and you're immediately hit with informational vertigo. Shelves littered with specialized fitness publications stretch into the distance, straining under the weight of the latest trends, fads and gimmicks. Head to the Web and you find more of the same. Those who are looking to simply trim a few inches off of their waistline or add a little muscle to their frame quickly become discouraged—not knowing which route is best, they rationalize that it is perhaps easier to never begin. Fitness, sadly, is one instance where the availability of info can be more a hindrance than a help.

The plain truth is that you don't need an expensive trainer, a pricey gym membership or even a subscription to an industry magazine. It is, as ever, about simplicity, consistency, progression and effort. Put those fundamentals together, as we do in *PrayFit,* and your body will respond in kind.

So go with your gut, because we've got your back. You've stepped over the line; the decision has been made. It's time to get PrayFit.

Simplicity

The best type of exercise is the kind that you will continue to do. And right at the top of the list for exercise that you will not continue to do is the complicated kind. No one sticks to a scheme that is replete with so many twists, turns and techniques that it's hard to keep it all straight. The good news is that you don't have to. Basic bodyweight movements use plenty of musculature, building a solid groundwork of strength for whatever goals you may have beyond these 28 to 56 days. *PrayFit* walks you through a basic, easy-to-follow routine that you can do in your living room—with zero equipment and even less hassle.

Consistency

People think that you have to perform some kind of activity every day to start effecting change in your appearance, health and vitality. While that's ideal, it's not entirely true. On this program, we'll ask you to challenge yourself physically four days per week—Monday, Tuesday, Thursday and Friday—for four weeks. Looking at it that way, you are only exercising 16 days out of a month. If you'd like to infuse other activity into your calendar over the course of these 28 to 56 days, be our guest. But the prescribed, bare-bones program laid out here will be plenty for you to handle if you're going full steam, particularly if you're new to exercise or are returning from a long layoff.

Progression

There is no understating the importance of progression when it comes to changing the body. You must remember: The body will only change to the level it is stressed. Loosely translated: If you keep challenging yourself, your body will keep getting stronger, fitter, leaner and faster. The *PrayFit* program revolves around daily progression. During each workout, you'll aim to beat your previous results, both in total reps and in time. For example, if in yesterday's workout, you completed 10 incline push-ups, 20 bodyweight squats and 30 crunches in, say, 5 minutes and 32 seconds, you'd want to do at least 11 incline push-ups, 21 bodyweight squats and 31 crunches in today's workout—in under 5 minutes and 32 seconds. And each week will build on the week before by adding new exercises and additional rounds of work. (For an illustration of how this works, see page 26.)

Effort

Your best effort today is your baseline goal for the next. Each workout is a chance to build on what you did last time. You'd be surprised what you can do when you strive for "just one more." The body, you'll remember, is the Lord's handiwork, and while we are each uniquely crafted, we all have enormous capacity to give a greater effort in all we do. This all-out attack on your previous best will keep you motivated and accountable. And when you start to see the reps climbing and your times falling, you'll be thankful you didn't hold anything back. Besides, these workouts are all very short in nature—likely topping out at 20 to 30 minutes for most people by the final week—so every second, every rep is even more valuable. Remember: Halfhearted efforts will, without fail, produce halfhearted results.

For video demonstrations of these exercises and others, visit www.prayfit.com/fitness.

PRAYFIT
Training Program Highlights

Manifest Density
Density training is simply packing more work into less time with each workout. This necessitates a personal insistence on progression each week.

Positive Failure
Keeping track of how many reps you should be doing is easy—just do as many as possible. This is called muscle failure—the point at which you can no longer complete the exercise with good form. Once you hit failure, stop, chart your number and move quickly to the next exercise.

Train Weaknesses First
Because legs are generally a strong body part, they are trained late or last. Upper body exercises will go first, when you are at your strongest.

No Specific Cardio
No treadmills or interval runs in this program. The pace at which you are performing these workouts will provide the aerobic stimulus you need to start burning fat.

Time Matters
Start your timing on the first rep and don't stop until your last.

Watch Rest; Don't Dwell on It
In weeks 2 to 4, when you're doing multiple rounds of a workout, you're free to rest between rounds—just know that the clock is ticking. Be honest with the clock and strive to reduce your rest times each workout. Note your rest in the journal space provided and try to shorten those rest periods from workout to workout.

Provides a Foundation
The bump you'll receive in strength, endurance and athleticism on this program will open doors to new forms of exercise, or for a return to this program with a better base to work from.

Each page will feature the following:

1. **The Workout:** A simple, straightforward roadmap to the day's activity. To the right of the workout, you'll have space to chart that day's total reps, as well as the time it took you to complete the exercises in the order listed. (For video demonstrations of these exercises and others, visit www.prayfit.com/fitness.)

2. **Firm Believer:** A tip or two that will help you continue to make progress. This will include an explanation of terms and concepts that you should familiarize yourself with to get the most out of the program.

3. **Food Byte:** Just what it says—a nutritional nugget of wisdom that you can pocket for the 28 days of this program and beyond. A full overview on nutrition can be found on page 205.

4. **PrayFit Recipe of the Week:** These recipes will be provided each week, helping you add spice and health to your nutritional repertoire. For more great recipes, visit prayfit.com.

5. **Journal Space:** You can use this area to scribble important information about that day's workout, such as how you felt, what was easy or hard, how you'd like to approach the next workout differently. You'll definitely want to note your rest periods. Or maybe you have a question you'd like to put to the PrayFit team? Write it here so you don't forget.

While privacy is one of the potential perks of this stay-at-home brand of fitness, the *PrayFit* plan is also great for small groups, couples or friends to work through together. These types of arrangements lend themselves to fantastic fellowship opportunities where participants can meet for Bible study and discuss physical fitness, and encourage each other in both.

Even if the *PrayFit* program is not your traditional mode of training— perhaps you're a runner or cyclist or simply an avid walker—its progression structure lends itself well to most active pursuits by providing increased strength, aerobic capacity and general overall performance.

Make this the start of something special. One month, 28 days. And if you can do one month, you'll find that the second (and third and fourth) is easier. God gave us these magnificent bodies; let's start using them to their full potential so that others may follow our example. We are lamps in a dark world—how is your commitment to your health lighting the way for others?

In Jesus' name, we train.

Journal Mandate

Writing down your results each day in the *PrayFit* program is no accident. Journaling is one of the most valuable yet underused tools of meeting and exceeding fitness goals. Keeping track of what you have done is essential if you expect to continue to make progress. Consider it a failsafe accountability system that pushes you toward your best body ever, in daily, quantifiable doses. To start your own online journal, or to view journals from other *PrayFit* readers, visit prayfit.com/forums.

SAMPLE FIT JOURNAL

Exercise	Reps Goal	Reps Rd. 1	Reps Rd. 2	Reps Total (2 Rounds)
Plyo push-up	17	11	9	20
Bodyweight squat	42	22	21	43
Crunch	37	25	24	49
Reverse crunch	29	20	15	35
Rd. time	9:25	4:00	5:05	9:05

At the start of each week, you'll be given a brand-new set of exercises. In the above example, you have the plyo push-up, bodyweight squat, crunch and reverse crunch. Yesterday's total performance on those exercises is indicated in the first column of the chart as the "goal" for today. You have to beat that number of reps; however, you also have the total time it took you to perform that many reps yesterday, seen at the bottom of the first column as "round time." So you also have to beat that time.

In this example workout, you're doing these exercises twice. So do the first round (Rd 1) of the plyo push-up to failure (until you can't perform another plyo push-up with good form) and write that number in the space. Then immediately begin the bodyweight squat, again working to failure. Write that number down; then the crunch, and so on. When you can't perform another rep of the last exercise on the list, in this case it's the crunch, you'll note those reps and then stop the clock (or simply note the time).

Taking as little rest as necessary, you will then begin the sequence again, beginning with the plyo push-up until you've gone all the way through the exercises a second time. The combined score of your two rounds of work totals go in the "Total" space on the right.

As each week goes on, your daily goal is to do more reps in less time each day than you were able to do previously. Then when the new week rolls around, the slate is clean and you'll be given a new set of exercises. Each new week's workout will be indicated by the words "Baseline Workout of the Week," and on each day you'll simply carry over your best numbers to become the new goals you'll strive to beat each day.

And finally, because the *PrayFit* program utilizes just your bodyweight, it's for anyone at any fitness level. The program is all relative.

Your best is not anybody else's best. So if you can do 25 total push-ups where someone else can only do 10 push-ups, that's fine. As long as each of you does at least one more the next time, in less time, you've done the task at hand. So whether you're an experienced athlete, a beginner or someone coming off of an injury or from years of layoff, this bodyweight-only plan will work for you.

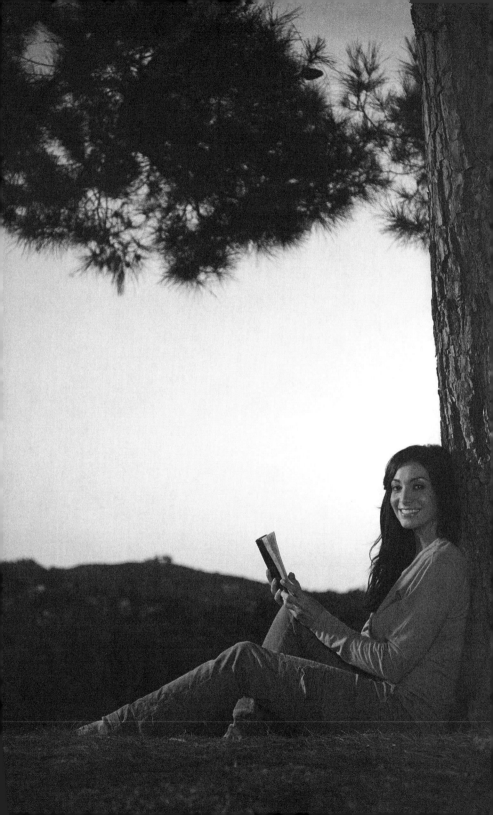

Month One

Decision Day:
28 Days to Fitness

Perhaps you've just awakened. The sun isn't even up. Your spouse is asleep and lying on his or her side; your kids are tucked tightly in their beds down the hall. It's just you.

You're about to hit your knees to hear from the Lord and to share your thoughts with Him about the day ahead.

Then you'll go from your knees to the floor, challenging yourself to become a physically renewed child of God. Not to be a mountain of muscle or a picture of perfection, but rather just a healthier person, spiritually and physically.

It's time to get up. It's time to be obedient.

It's time to PrayFit.

We can be tired, weary and emotionally distraught,
but after spending time alone with God, we find that He injects
into our bodies energy, power and strength.

DR. CHARLES STANLEY

Extreme Makeover: Heart Edition

Faith
The Exercise: 2 Corinthians 5

Last year, I had the privilege of spending a week on the set of ABC's *Extreme Makeover: Home Edition*. When it finally aired on television, I remembered the feeling I had when that family first answered the knock at the door, then came back a week later to a brand-new house. Talk about gut wrenching! Someone they never expected came into their world and freely gave them something they couldn't afford on their own. He saw where they lived and said you don't have to live here anymore.

As I watched the process, I couldn't help but think of Jesus. Just like we did for that family, He knocks gently, anxiously awaiting our answer. But instead of calling for a wrecking ball, He does the unthinkable: He moves in. Instead of a hammer, He carries a suitcase. He gives us something we could never afford on our own—Himself—telling us we don't have to live here anymore, alone.

—Peña

Pastor's Point

1. Getting a new start is such a gift. By putting our faith in Jesus, we don't just get a new start—we get a new life—forever.
2. What parts of the "old you" are still hanging on? Old thoughts? Old attitudes? Old emotions?
3. What areas of your character does God still need to reconstruct?
4. Additional reading: Galatians 2:20.

Today's Prayer

Lord, You are the only one who can tear down the old nature and replace it with the new—forever. My body will break down, my home will need repair, but Your makeover of my heart and mind and spirit is permanent. Thank You for making me new.

Walking with Him

The gift that Jesus offers us is an "extreme makeover." But this makeover doesn't make bad people into good people; it transforms dead people into people who will live forever. When you believe in Jesus—that He is the Son of God who died for your sins and rose again to give you eternal life—you are given a new home; you are part of God's family. Have you put your faith in Jesus?

Fitness
Workout #1: Baseline, Week 1

Training at a Glance

Today is your first session of scheduled exercise with *PrayFit*. What an exciting undertaking! But don't let the simplicity of today's workout, or any other in this book, numb you into thinking that it will be a walk in the park. In order to get the most out of this program, do as many reps as possible using good form on each exercise.

Exercise	Reps
Incline push-up	
Crunch	
Rd. time	

Before you begin the exercises, warm up by walking or jogging in place for three to five minutes. Your goal is to perform a total of at least one more rep than you did in your last workout, on each exercise and in less total time.

Exercises of the Week

Incline Push-Up
Focus: Lower Chest, Shoulders, Back, Abs

Find a wall, a sturdy end of a couch or a flat bench and place your hands against it wider than shoulder-width apart. With your feet stable a couple of feet behind you, press until your arms are fully extended. Flex and squeeze your chest, shoulders and arms at the top then slowly lower yourself to the start. When your chest reaches an inch or so away from the stable platform, press yourself up again and repeat.

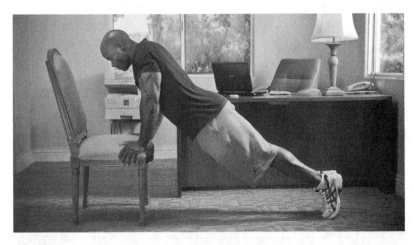

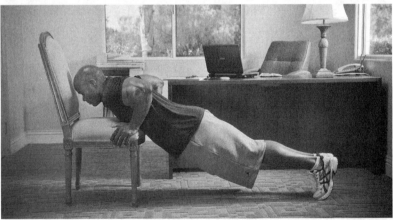

Crunch
Focus: Upper Abs

Lie face-up on the floor with your hands cupped gently behind your head (do not pull on your neck). Keeping your knees bent and with your feet flat on the floor, crunch your upper body up until your shoulder blades are off the floor. Squeeze your abs, then lower yourself back to the start and repeat.

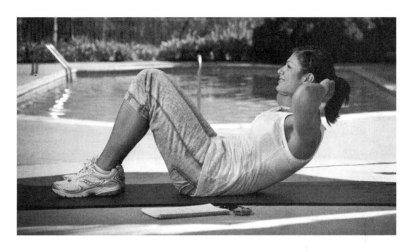

Firm Believer

You know the push-up. It's a stalwart exercise that's stood the test of time. You would think it would be hard to improve upon such a classic— and you'd be right. The incline version prescribed here isn't meant to be better, just different. Depending on the variation you choose—wall, couch, and so forth—the move will stimulate the muscles of your chest, shoulders and arms differently. (For video demonstrations of the exercises used in this book, visit www.prayfit.com/fitness.)

Food Byte

Macronutrients are the classes of chemical compounds humans consume in the largest quantities and that provide bulk energy. These are protein, fat and carbohydrate.

Marching Orders

Faith
The Exercise: Joshua 6

Joshua could have related to our steep challenges. His neck cramped as he surveyed the impregnable wall of Jericho. "Gonna need a bigger army," he whispered out of the side of his mouth. You might be saying the same about your predicament. Does something at school or work have you hoping for reinforcements? If so, stand next to Joshua as he listens to God's strategy.

"Then on the seventh day you shall march around the city seven times, and the priests shall blow the trumpets . . . and the wall of the city will fall down flat" (Josh. 6:4-5).

"That's it? That's the plan?" this time those words come out of the side of *your* mouth. I wonder if Joshua paused when he heard the order. After all, he was among men of war (v. 3) and probably dressed for the occasion. I'm not sure if he hesitated when he got his orders, but I know we sure do. When we have to respect a less than respectful boss, or when it seems the rules only apply to us, obeying God's marching orders is sometimes the last thing we want to do (or actually do), especially if we're ready to fight.

But we all know the story. Joshua's army walked around Jericho for seven days without making a sound or saying a word. Then, when it was time, they blew the trumpets, shouted, and the walls came tumbling down. God's enemies might have laughed and scoffed for a week, but being obedient has never proven to be popular or easy, just effective.

So the next time we feel like taking the wall ourselves, let's wait with Joshua. He listened, walked without talking and then praised God on day seven. Sooner or later, like Jericho, the world will see we're not just walking in circles.

—Peña

Pastor's Point

1. Has it ever seemed like God's plans couldn't possibly be right? Like He made a mistake?
2. Do you have a hard time obeying God when it might appear foolish to others? Why or why not?

Today's Prayer

Lord, sometimes the plans You have seem foolish to everybody else, but I will trust in You. Help me to wait patiently for Your plan to be clear.

Walking with Him

God loves to make things look impossible or even a little bit foolish. In the Bible account, from Gideon to Joshua to the Red Sea to talking donkeys, God created situations that would be impossible without Him. He does the same today. That way, we can never take the credit when it all works out. Put your trust in God, especially when it seems like all hope has been lost.

Fitness
Workout #2

Training at a Glance

It should look familiar, the incline push-up followed by the crunch. But remember, you're building a foundation of fitness, so attack each training session with vigor, because the benefit lies in how you improve over time. Do each rep with energy, passion and a desire to improve on your previous session, and it's guaranteed you'll get the most from your efforts.

Exercise	Reps Goal	Reps Rd. 1	Total
Incline push-up			
Crunch			
Rd. time			

Before you begin the exercises, warm up by walking or jogging in place for three to five minutes. Your goal is to perform a total of at least one

more rep than you did in your last workout on each exercise and in less total time.

Firm Believer

Always warm up. And, yes, this comes before stretching (since we won't stretch until after the workout). Get blood flowing to your muscles and joints through some simple dynamic movements such as jumping jacks or walking/running in place. This will help to prep your body for the work that is ahead.

Food Byte

A high-protein diet not only promotes lean body mass, but it also enhances fat loss. Researchers at Skidmore College found that when subjects followed a high-protein diet for eight weeks, they lost significantly more body fat, particularly abdominal fat, than those following a low-fat/high-carb diet.

Hearing from God

Faith
The Exercise: 1 Kings 19:9-12

Sometimes the hectic pace of life is deafening. The alarm sounds, the day starts and we hit the ground running. The thought of taking time to enter the day on our knees is almost uncomfortable because the list of to-dos is waiting, the clock is ticking, and the schedule has begun.

We race from one activity to the next and ask God to bless our work, to be with us, to keep up. We reason that God will understand because He knows the mountain of responsibilities that we face. But it's absolutely impossible to hear God in the chaos of life. Elijah, one of God's great prophets, experienced this firsthand. He was used to hearing from God in a personal way. God spoke to Him in the quiet moments when he was not distracted. A great and powerful wind came, but God was not in the wind. Then came an earthquake and fire, but God was not there either. Finally, a gentle whisper came, and Elijah heard His voice.

I wonder if most of the time we just plain miss His presence because we don't slow down long enough or get quiet enough to hear. In Psalm 46:10, we are told to "Be still, and know that I am God."

Sometimes we expect God to be more obvious. We want Him to give us a sign. But God wants us to train our ear to hear His voice. He wants us to unplug from the email, the voicemail, the TV, the iPod and the Blackberry and actually appreciate silence. He wants our undivided attention so He can bring real transformation from the inside out. So start each day here, in your quiet place, and be still. If you listen for His voice He'll speak to your heart through His Word. Let Him probe your conscience and bring things to mind that need to be changed. He'll encourage you to dig deeper and stay the course. Your journey to a healthier life has begun.

—Page

1. In what ways has the pace of your life crowded out time for connection with God?
2. What time each day will you commit to spending quiet time to just listen, pray and read His Word?
3. Additional reading: Luke 5:16; Mark 1:35.

Today's Prayer

Lord, I pray that I would slow down long enough to be still and know that You are God. Give me the desire and the discipline to start my day first with You so that I may hear Your voice.

Walking with Him

Schedule time with the Lord. Over the course of a day, it is so easy to fit in meetings, meals and workouts; but rarely do we "pencil in" a set time for the Lord (except for 9:00 or 11:00 on Sunday mornings, perhaps). So pick a time and stick to it. As with exercise, consistency is the key to spiritual growth.

Fitness
Rest

Fitness in Focus: Your First Rest Day. Throughout the next 28 days, you'll need plenty of good rest, especially because you'll be taking each one of your workouts to the limit. So we've built in rest days to help you recover physically and mentally. You might already know that it's during rest periods following strenuous exercise that our bodies get stronger, fitter, leaner. After they repair, they can handle more work, more stress. And as you progress in the plan, these rest days will be more and more appreciated.

On your rest days, you're welcome to perform other fun activities—like cardiovascular training, such as going for a walk or bike ride—but we suggest you rest from the bodyweight exercises within the program and especially any resistance-type of activities. This will allow your body the necessary recovery time it needs to be at its best for the next few days of activity.

However, even though we want you to rest your body on days 3, 6 and 7 of each week, we still want you to train your mind. For that reason, on your rest days we'll accompany your devotion with some health and fitness information you might not have known. From anatomy, physiology and nutrition, you'll complete *PrayFit* not only more fit, but you'll also have a better understanding of the body and how it responds to exercise. It is a true daily mind, body and soul experience.

According to the CDC, one-third of U.S. adults are obese, and the latest population-level data indicate no reversal of the upward trend.

4

You Have a
Friend Request

Faith
The Exercise: Jeremiah 31:34

I'm fairly new to Facebook. I'm amazed to see the faces and the old, familiar places that once were on the tip of my tongue. Stomping-ground buddies (and bullies) are now hardworking husbands and tenderhearted dads. And with each new friend request comes a flood of memories—for me, two in particular.

I was maybe six or seven, and I had just figured out that there was no Santa Claus. Boy, was I mad. I ran outside, and the first person I told was my next-door neighbor. She was maybe four years old . . . oh yeah, you bet I told her! It was time for kids to unite! Long story short, I got in major trouble. Thing is, recently on Facebook, I reunited with my young neighbor and, wouldn't you know it, she doesn't remember that at all. Lesson number one.

Later, in college, I decided that I was too cool to have a roommate, so I forced my way to a private dorm room, leaving behind a friend who needed me. To this day, it's one of my biggest regrets. I can't believe my heart, and I can't fathom why I acted that way. I reached out to him recently as well, and though I wouldn't blame him if he didn't, he forgave me completely. Lesson number two.

Two friends, one request. One completely forgot. The other completely forgave. Reminds me of another who does both.

—Peña

Pastor's Point

1. Are there things in your past for which you have trouble forgiving yourself?
2. What do you think about the fact that the Lord has a short memory for your sin?
3. Additional reading: Matthew 6:14-15; 18:21-22.

Today's Prayer

Lord, I am a broken sinner. I do things, say things and think things on a daily basis that I know do not please You. I pray that You would forgive my sins and that You would help me turn away from my sinful nature.

Walking with Him

It's time to get honest and real. Each one of us struggles with sins that are tougher than others—those that we struggle with on a daily basis. Be honest with yourself and the Lord about what those sins are and take active, measurable steps to eliminate them today.

Fitness
Workout #3

Training at a Glance

How are you doing so far on your crunches? Do they burn right down to your core? If not, you'll want to push harder. You see, there are few things more painful than the muscle burn you build in your abs; but on the other hand, it's that feeling that indicates you are challenging the muscles of your midsection and making yourself stronger. Learn to embrace the burn.

Exercise	Reps Goal	Reps Rd. 1	Total
Incline push-up			
Crunch			
Rd. time			

Before you begin the exercises, warm up by walking or jogging in place for three to five minutes. Your goal is to perform a total of at least one

more rep than you did in your last workout on each exercise and in less total time.

Firm Believer

Be sure to cool down. Following a workout, it's important to slowly bring your muscles back from the brink. A walk around the house should suffice to shuttle waste products out of your muscles and bring your heart rate back down gradually.

Food Byte

Fruits and vegetables contain compounds known as antioxidants. These naturally occurring substances help protect cells all over the body from damage; they also combat inflammation and help you look and feel fabulous. As a rule of thumb, the brighter the color of the fruit, the more antioxidants it possesses.

Come What May

Faith
The Exercise: Romans 8:38-39

If you're like me, you started the week with huge goals. Finding a goldmine was the least of your objectives. And conquering the world? Only the beginning. Just for fun, you thought you'd punch out the moon as well. And so, with a little hop in your step, you whistled "Come What May" on your way out the door.

But what came your way was anything but anticipated. Instead, you were ambushed with issues, blindsided by problems and drilled in the gut with unwanted surprises. Things just didn't go as planned, to say nothing about finding that goldmine. Today, finding your car keys will do just fine.

But underneath the week's rubble is one sure promise, a very certain truth. God never leaves us. He never forsakes us. Though it seemed like you fell a thousand feet, coming close to hitting rock bottom, God never loosened His grasp. You're as much in His strong, protective grip today as you were on Monday. His love is stronger, and His grace is deeper, wider and higher than anything that tried to steal your joy.

So let's finish the week together. And while we might be limping from a fall or two—not to mention this week's workouts—our song of praise can still echo. But in my case, instead of humming "Come What May," I think I'll go with "Amazing Grace."

—Peña

Pastor's Point

1. How do you respond when you have one of those days when nothing seems to go right?
2. What might God be trying to reveal and refine in you through the trials?
3. Additional reading: Ephesians 3:16-21; James 1:2-4.

Today's Prayer

Lord, Your love is amazing. The fact that it is constant, unwavering and unending is sometimes too much to grasp. Help me, Lord, to be an extension of Your love for me in the world.

Walking with Him

Love others as the Lord loves us—without conditions and without limit. Though loving in this fashion may make us vulnerable, it is the only way the Lord would have us do it. His love reflected through our lives, and the way we love others, is a great heavenly net to cast into the world.

Fitness
Workout #4

Training at a Glance

You may think the strength of your muscles is the limiting factor in how many reps you can complete—but that's not necessarily the case. Your mind plays a key part. As you do your reps, try to find the zone: Focus on your breathing and the rhythm of each rep, and you'll find yourself pumping out more pure, clean reps than you may have thought possible.

Exercise	Reps Goal	Reps Rd. 1	Total
Incline push-up			
Crunch			
Rd. time			

Before you begin the exercises, warm up by walking or jogging in place for three to five minutes. Your goal is to perform a total of at least one

more rep than you did in your last workout on each exercise and in less total time.

Firm Believer

Know when to stretch. A common misconception is that you should stretch before your workout. This is not only dangerous—trying to stretch cold muscles is like trying to stretch a sun-dried rubber band—but it can actually temporarily reduce strength in those muscles, making it a bad idea for a pre-workout ritual.

Food Byte

Protein from fish, poultry and lean cuts of beef are ideal sources for muscle repair and maintenance; but don't count out plant proteins like beans, soy and dairy. Incorporate these protein powerhouses into most meals to keep your muscles fueled and fit.

Overcoming Doubts and Fears

Faith
The Exercise: 1 Samuel 17

So many of us are absolutely paralyzed by fear. We continually remind ourselves of our weaknesses, limitations and past failures. Sometimes the obstacles are real and sometimes they just appear to be real. Either way, doubts and fears often rob us of experiencing God's power and presence in the midst of our circumstances.

We have been made in the likeness of Almighty God. And yet we seem to believe the lies of the enemy—that we can't do it, that we have failed and we will fail again.

The entire nation of Israel, God's chosen, was frozen by fear. For 40 days, taunts rained down on their camp every morning and every evening from a giant of unequalled physical stature. Goliath mocked the very God that had faithfully delivered His people against oppressive enemies. But no response came from the Israelites, even when Saul promised his daughter and great wealth to the one who could kill the giant. They let doubts and defeat enter their minds and even their hearts. No one would rise to the challenge—except David. The Scripture tells us that David, just a teenager, "ran to the battle lines." David heard the giant's challenge and saw the soldiers' fear firsthand. He was then reminded that he was just a boy—that he was too little and too young to fight the giant.

But David would have none of it; he kept his eyes on the size of his God, not the size of the giant. And that is our lesson—when we focus on our own weaknesses or failures, doubt and fear will bring defeat. But when we focus on God and His power and faithfulness, we can overcome even our greatest challenge. By choosing to take this challenge and face your giants, you are like David. And when doubts and fears and negative thoughts rain down on you in the morning and in the evening, have none of it. Take every thought captive. Eliminate negative thinking. Replace it with Scripture and speak it out loud. You will encounter challenges along this journey, but you will overcome them! Trust Him to deepen your faith and revitalize your health.

—Page

Pastor's Point

1. In what ways have you let doubts and fears prevent you from taking risks and attempting great things for God?
2. "Listen" to your thoughts today and turn all of the negative into positive.
3. Additional reading: Isaiah 40:10-13; Luke 12:4-5.

Today's Prayer

Lord, I pray that I will focus not on my past failures or weaknesses, or even on my current challenges, but that I will put my trust in Your power to face my giants and overcome my doubts and fears.

Walking with Him

Realize that while you are broken and will stumble, the Lord is always there to pick you up. Past failure? Let it go. Insecurity about your ability to do great things? Set it aside. Make it your task today to inject more positivity into your daily walk.

Fitness
Rest

Fitness in Focus: Journaling. It's virtually impossible to remember all the exercises or details of a particular workout from one day to the next. That's why keeping a journal is so important to your health and fitness goals. Seeing yesterday's best as today's quest is how to make sure you're making progress.

Along with your pen or pencil, have a stopwatch at hand. The stopwatch is especially important if you train at home. Keeping the watch right next to the journal will help you immediately track your time and reps, rather than looking for the clock. Each day and week, you'll have more exercises and improvement in performance, and your time and reps will be your markers for such progress.

Here's a list of what you should aim to track with each workout:

1. **Rest periods:** How long you take between circuits—and how much less is needed from week to week—can help you track how fit you are becoming.

2. **Fatigue:** Did you feel lethargic or energetic as you went through your workout? Knowing which one it is can help you determine if there are other factors to consider such as your sleep schedule, diet or warm-up.

3. **Diet:** Make it a habit to list what you ate leading up to to-day's workout. Didn't have time to eat? Chart that and compare it to workouts where you were able to get some nutritious foods in ahead of time.

4. **Performance:** How would you grade yourself? Were there some movements that you were better at than others? Where do you need improvement? This more broad-based category can help you identify and snuff out weaknesses.

To start your own digital workout journal, visit www.prayfit.com/forum.

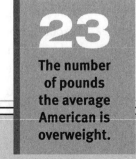

23

The number of pounds the average American is overweight.

The Word Walks

Faith
The Exercise: John 1:1-34

When I stop to think about the fact that God, the Creator of the entire universe, actually humbled Himself to become like us and walk with us on the earth, it's hard to even get my head around it.

His humility is staggering.

The Creator of everything that we see (and even the stuff that we have yet to see) came as a man, took on the limits of time and space, and willingly laid down His life so that we could live with Him forever. Amazing.

His love is immeasurable.

All at once I am aware that God cared enough about me that He would "walk in my shoes" so that I would know that He was acquainted with my real-life struggle and pain and joy.

His sacrifice is complete.

And when I realize that Jesus already knew the road that He would walk would end at the cross of Calvary—that He would be betrayed, beaten, ridiculed, humiliated and eventually crucified by those that He made, loved and had come to save—I realize my own need of the Savior.

Jesus walked on earth so that those of us who would receive Him and believe in His name would be given the right to be called children of God. Now that is a priceless gift.

—Page

Pastor's Point

1. What does John 1 reveal about who Jesus is and what He did?
2. What happens when we receive Jesus and believe in His name (see vv. 12-13)? Why is this important?
3. Additional reading: Acts 4:12; Philippians 2:5-8.

Today's Prayer

Lord, I thank You that Jesus, the very Creator of what is seen and unseen, willingly stepped out of heaven and became man. Thank You for giving me the right to be called Your child as I put my faith in Jesus.

Walking with Him

Acknowledge what the Lord did for you. Revisit the scene in your mind. It's easy to lose sight of what happened to Jesus in His final hours. You may be aware of the Lord's presence or His work in your life, but you can sometimes forget the magnitude of what Jesus went through and accomplished for you on the cross. He washed your sins clean with the blood of His only begotten Son. Use the space below to jot down your visceral reaction to Jesus' crucifixion. How does it make you feel? What does it say about the price He paid to make you His?

PrayFit Recipe of the Week
Pineapple-Berry Smoothie

½ cup sliced strawberries
¾ cup diced pineapple
¼ cup plain, low-fat yogurt
1 scoop vanilla whey protein powder
Water
Crushed ice

Place ingredients in a blender and blend until smooth.

Calories: 222 | **Protein:** 28 grams | **Carbohydrates:** 28 grams | **Fat:** 1 gram

A Hopeful Monday

Faith
The Exercise: Luke 5:5-11

Peter would know about Mondays.

Well, he would have known how you feel on Mondays. In our Luke 5 passage of Scripture, he's just come home after working an all-nighter, and he's tired. Add to that the fact that he has nothing to show for his labor and you could say he's short on funds and maybe shorter on patience. The last thing he wants to do is turn the boat around and head back out. But in this passage, that's exactly what Jesus asks him to do.

"Master, we worked all night and caught nothing, but if you say so, I'll lower the nets," he says to Jesus, who is standing on the shore.

Thankfully, Peter had more discipline than optimism, because he ended up catching more than fish.

Do you feel like you are in Peter's boat? Is your week ahead looking more like a shallow lake than a sea of opportunity? Are you heading back to the same job, the same boss, the same staff, knowing that what lies ahead is much of the same? Well, do what Peter did. Try the other side of the boat. Try a different approach, a different style. And as you cast your *line of work* into the week, take a backward glance at the shore to see Jesus grinning at today's success.

Let's turn the boat around and catch the week by surprise, shall we?

—Peña

Pastor's Point

1. What kind of mood will you take into this coming Monday?
2. What does Peter's submission to Jesus say about the results of trusting the Lord?
3. Additional reading: John 14:23; Acts 5:29-32.

Today's Prayer

Lord, I may not always understand what You are leading me to do, so help me to simply trust that You know what is best for me. Help me go deeper in my walk with You.

Walking with Him

Jesus always wants us to dig deeper; He is never satisfied when we stay on the surface, because He knows that the biggest fish always swim in the deepest waters. Can you go deeper in your relationship with Him? What will it take? More time? More listening? More trusting?

Fitness
Workout #5: Baseline, Week 2

Training at a Glance

A gut check (literally, in fact)—are you doing your crunches too quickly? When focused on beating a number, it can get tempting to blast through your crunches at lightning speed, especially because the whole PrayFit workout strategy is designed around doing more work in less time. While speed may be a benefit in some dynamic forms of exercise, when it comes to abs, slow and steady wins the day. Today, try counting two seconds to raise (one-one thousand, two-one thousand), and two to three seconds down to find a more potent cadence, which will also help you set a more viable baseline.

Before you begin the exercises, warm up by walking or jogging in place for three to five minutes. Your goal is to perform a total of at least one more rep than you did in your last workout on each exercise and in less total time.

Exercise	Reps Goal	Reps Rd. 1	Reps Rd. 2	Reps Total (2 Rounds)
Standard push-up*				
Bodyweight squat*				
Crunch				
Rd. time				

*New exercise

New Exercises of the Week

Standard Push-Up or Modified Push-up from the Knees

Focus: Chest, shoulders, back, abs

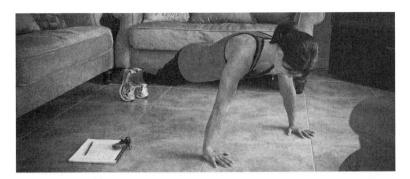

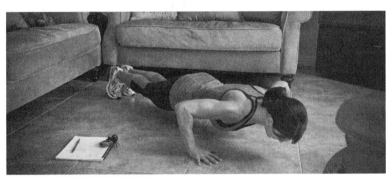

Get into a push-up position with your body in a straight line (or on your knees), feet together, hands wider than shoulder-width apart and your eyes focused on the floor. Press yourself up to full arm extension, keeping your abs tight and back straight. Squeeze your arms and chest at the top, then lower yourself to the start and repeat. Don't bounce your chest off the floor, but rather start each rep when your chest reaches a point an inch or so away from the floor.

Bodyweight Squat

Focus: Legs, glutes, hamstrings, lower back

Stand with your feet about shoulder-width apart, a light bend in your knees and your toes turned out slightly. Keeping your head neutral, abs tight and torso erect, bend at the knees and hips to slowly lower your body as if you were going to sit down in a chair. Pause when your legs reach a 90-degree angle, and then forcefully drive through your heels, extending at your hips and knees until you arrive at the standing position.

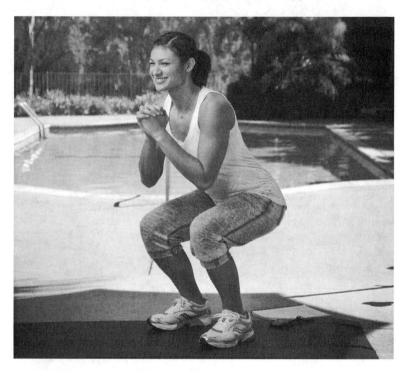

Firm Believer

Always take each set of exercises to failure. In other words, don't simply pick a number of push-ups or ab moves and stop at that number, because it doesn't do your body any good to stop at, say, 25 reps, when you could have done 35. So remember, because your own weight is the resistance, take each set to exhaustion.

Food Byte

Not only will certain fats not lead to fat gain, but they can actually lead to fat loss. Eating fat to lose fat seems counterintuitive, but if you keep your fat intake around 30 percent of your total daily calories, as prescribed in the *Pray-Fit* nutrition plan, you can actually boost your fat loss compared to eating a low-fat diet. Choose foods like fatty fish, nuts, olive oil and peanut butter.

Unload the Burden

Faith
The Exercise: Matthew 11:28

I was in the eighth grade when I first came to know the Lord. After church on Sunday, in a corner of my bedroom, I got down on my knees and asked Jesus into my heart and life.

But over the course of that year, I kept it quiet. I'm not sure if I was uncertain or embarrassed or both, but what had happened in my heart stayed hidden there. Doubt started to creep in. Was I really saved? How could I be sure? Is there even a God? It seemed like my prayers went as high as the ceiling.

Then one day at church, my heart was so troubled that I decided to walk the aisle. During the closing song, I went down front, got down on one knee and started to pray. Then a sweet, elderly man whose voice I didn't recognize and whose face I never saw, put his hand on my shoulder and whispered words I'll never forget. He said, "Son, when you come to the cross, whatever you're carrying or whatever is bothering you, just lay it down right there. And when you get up, leave it there. Give it to Jesus, and walk away." He removed his hand from my shoulder and I stayed there in a flood of eighth-grade tears. But when I stood, that burden was gone.

You know, I never found out who that man was. But he had more of an impact on my life than he'll ever know. Do you know of someone like that? Maybe he or she was that kind of encouragement to you. Perhaps you've been that someone for others. Whichever the case, there are those around us who are hurting—financially, socially, physically—you name it. Lots of people are walking their own private aisles in need of a hand, a voice and a Savior.

—Peña

Pastor's Point

1. When you come to the cross, do you truly set your burdens down? Or do you take them with you when you leave?
2. Do you know if you've ever made a profound impact on someone's faith? If so, how did that make you feel?
3. Additional reading: 1 Peter 5:6-7; Psalm 55:22.

Today's Prayer

Lord, I carry so much on my shoulders each day. I know that You want us to lay our burdens at the foot of the cross, but sometimes it's difficult. Lord, help me have the faith to leave them with You and to remember that I can walk away knowing that You are God and that Your Son died to lighten my burdens.

Walking with Him

Give thanks to the Lord, not just for your salvation, but also for the people in your life that He has used along the way to help you grow in your faith. An encouraging word to someone who has lent you a hand and a voice in the past could find them in need of that spiritual boost.

Fitness
Workout #6

Training at a Glance

Last week, you did the incline push-up, which, as we mentioned, is not better than the standard version—just different. So it should be no surprise that the standard military style push-up made its debut this week, thus slightly altering the area of stimulation from your lower pecs to the middle region of the muscle.

Exercise	Reps Goal	Reps Rd. 1	Reps Rd. 2	Reps Total (2 Rounds)
Standard push-up				
Bodyweight squat				
Crunch				
Rd. time				

Before you begin the exercises, warm up by walking or jogging in place for three to five minutes. Your goal is to perform a total of at least one more rep than you did in your last workout on each exercise and in less total time.

Firm Believer

Finding a partner to exercise with is one of the best things you can do to reach your fitness goals. Having a partner breeds accountability because you're far less likely to skip a workout if you know someone is counting on you. It provides competition since even the least competitive person hates to be outdone on a regular basis. Just make sure you pick a partner who is as serious about getting fit as you are.

Food Byte

Heart-healthy omega-3 fats are found in fatty fish like salmon, tuna and sardines. In addition to the heart benefits, these fats play an important role in growth and brain function.

Make a Decision

Faith
The Exercise: Daniel 1:8

Talk is cheap, isn't it? Think about how many resolutions are made and broken within weeks of the initial commitment. We all have good intentions, but somehow our resolve fades over time and we fall back into our failed patterns of behavior that have robbed us of the fullness of life Jesus came to give. So as we tackle this new challenge, as we pursue a deep relationship with God and abundant health, we do it with our eyes on the prize. Godliness never happens by accident. Nor does good health.

Daniel and his friends Hananiah, Mishael and Azariah were Israelites from the royal family. They were handsome, bright and quick to learn. They were considered the best of the best. And the Babylonian King Nebuchadnezzar wanted them; he put them into his training program designed to fully indoctrinate them into the ways and culture of Babylon. The culture was attractive and enticing. It appealed to one's desire for success, sensuality, self-indulgence and status. Sounds familiar, doesn't it?

But even though Daniel was surrounded by the allure of this culture, he resisted its pull and remained true to God. He would not eat the royal food offered to idols. And, he put God to the test. Lesser men would have crumbled under the pressure, but not Daniel. His decision to follow God was not one of convenience. It was a matter of consistency and loyalty. The decision to pursue God, to grow deep spiritual roots and to walk with God in a personal way requires resolve. Not the kind of resolve that is broken by excuses or obstacles.

And the great truth here is that it actually feels good to take a stand and do things differently. It produces courage, especially when you know that you have stood with God. And this courage then grows into an even greater resolve to follow through, overcome challenges and stay the course.

—Page

Pastor's Point

1. What actions can you take to do things differently than everybody else?
2. What are common ways that you give in to the pressure of those around you? With food? With lifestyle?
3. Additional reading: Daniel 3:16-18; 6:10-12.

Today's Prayer

Lord, I pray that I will choose to obey You, even when I'm not sure how it's going to turn out. I know that Your ways are always best and that You will produce great faith in me as I take my stand.

Walking with Him

Have you been seduced by a life of leisure, a life of convenience or the pursuit of affluence? Unfortunately, these things do not produce godliness. But by resolving to pursue spiritual depth and physical health, you can be like Daniel. Take a stand. Do life God's way.

Fitness
Rest

Fitness in Focus: Goal Building. Seeing all the way to the finish line from the starting gate can be difficult. The solution is to set smaller, more attainable goals—consider them rest stops on your route—that ultimately put you closer to where you want to be.

For many people, a new program accompanies a weight-loss goal. "I want to lose the 30 pounds I put on after college," someone might say. Well, that can be an intimidating number to reach. So instead of simply focusing on the 30 pounds, it may make more sense to lay out this type of plan:

By 2 weeks: 5 pounds
By 4 weeks: 10 pounds
By 6 weeks: 20 pounds
After 8 weeks: 25 pounds

Sure these are aggressive goals, but we're not messing around, are we? To accomplish great things, we have to set amazing goals. Perhaps these goals might even be out of reach, but it won't be due to a lack of striving.

What is your goal? Are you willing to put in the time to accomplish it?

$147 Billion

The amount spent by the U.S. annually on obesity-related health issues.

Deny the Flesh

Faith
The Exercise: Galatians 5:16-26

Have you ever seen anyone running on the treadmill while eating a bag of Cheetos? I recently witnessed one of my favorite pastors doing that very thing. Obviously, he couldn't keep up the workout for long. And while that idea may seem ridiculous, many of us are actually doing that very thing. We make some healthy choices, but we just don't want to give anything up. We want to have our cake and eat it too. In fact, many of us exercise just so we can eat whatever we want.

Blogs and weight-loss websites say to never deny yourself anything indefinitely. They say that when you're deprived of something you want, you're likely to crash and burn in a big way. Even billboards shout at us to "Eat what you crave." But this is not what God teaches. In Galatians 5 and Romans 8, we're told not to indulge in the sinful nature.

What's more, these Scripture passages tell us that it's impossible to live by the Spirit while satisfying the desires of the flesh. We won't get healthy by working out and then eating garbage, just like we won't live with God's power and produce fruit when we're engaged in gluttony or lust or anger or selfish ambition or jealousy or sexual immorality.

These things are in conflict with each other. The great news is that when you start to deny the flesh—deny your cravings and stop feeding yourself every single thing that you want—you actually live with power to overcome a lot of other struggles.

I've found that when I exercise self-control and abstain for a period of time from a food that I may really want—and if I set my mind on God and am filled with His Spirit—I actually enjoy victory physically as well as spiritually. The Spirit of God actually makes life more satisfying if we will simply resist temptations and pursue Him.

—Page

Pastor's Point

1. Are you readily giving in to certain cravings and desires?
2. Can you see the ways that this is hurting you as you walk with Christ?
3. Additional reading: Galatians 5:1-15; Romans 8:1-14.

Today's Prayer

Lord, I pray that You would empower me to overcome the desires of the sinful nature. I pray that You will fill me with Your Holy Spirit so that I can make choices that result in health and life.

Walking with Him

It's not easy to deny your cravings when everywhere you look is temptation. But just how different could your life look if you did? Would others ask where you get your strength to overcome? You bet they would. Name three cravings that you are willing to give up to grow.

Fitness
Workout #7

Training at a Glance

Because you are not using weight during the bodyweight squat, you may get tempted to become a little lax regarding your form. Don't do it—these early training sessions are forging the neural pathways through your body that will dictate how you move whenever you do a squat in the future. As you've heard, in many sports, from golf to baseball, it's easier to learn something correctly the first time than to unlearn bad habits later. Revisit the exercise how-tos and make sure you're following the instructions to the letter.

Before you begin the exercises, warm up by walking or jogging in place for three to five minutes. Your goal is to perform a total of at least one more rep than you did in your last workout on each exercise and in less total time.

Exercise	Reps Goal	Reps Rd. 1	Reps Rd. 2	Reps Total (2 Rounds)
Standard push-up				
Bodyweight squat				
Crunch				
Rd. time				

Firm Believer

A lot of people think that doing crunches all day will give you a set of six-pack abs. While training your abdominal muscles will definitely build strength in that region, it is your diet that is most responsible for that well-defined look. That's why you should try to avoid gimmicky fitness items that promise you better abs through exercise alone. Our *PrayFit* nutrition plan, combined with our high-intensity exercise, will help you get started on your way to a leaner midsection.

Food Byte

When it comes to dairy, choose nonfat or low-fat milk, yogurt and cheese. They have all the calcium and protein with a fraction of the saturated fat.

Play Ball, Dad's Here

Faith
The Exercise: John 10:27

Just as the Lord's sheep know His voice, I know my dad's whistle.

Growing up, I played lots of sports. I spent the majority of my after-noons at practice. In summer time and during the school year, after school, if I wasn't at home, I was probably on the field. Of all the things that stick out in my mind about practice, it's not the plays we ran or the opponents we prepared for. It was that moment that I knew my dad was near. See, my dad—like many dads—has a whistle that his boys know very well.

Each day, about halfway through practice, I'd hear it. A quick, sharp whistle; and even though it wasn't very loud, I could hear it through a hurricane. I'd turn, and in the corner of the field I'd see the familiar light blue shirt and dark pants. Yep, Dad was here.

He never missed a chance to cheer me on. And be it a practice or game day, when I heard that whistle, even though I couldn't always see him in the crowd, I was able to relax and play. Why? I think because that whistle meant so many things. A dad's whistle means, "I love you, my boy . . . hit that ball . . . and keep that chin up," all at the same time. And yep, it also meant that no matter what happened on the field, I knew he was taking me home.

As we practice this life, isn't it amazing to know that God is so close? He watches over us. He never misses a day to cheer us on. And we can play with confidence, knowing that when the game of life is over, He'll be there to take us home.

—Peña

Pastor's Point

1. Can you think of a time when you sought the Lord's guidance but weren't sure about His answer?
2. What can you do so you are better able to recognize His voice?
3. Additional reading: 1 Peter 2:25; John 21:15-17.

Today's Prayer

Lord, I hear You. Even in silence, Your answers to my prayers are perfectly clear. I know that when I seek You with all my heart I will find You and Your will for my life. Thank You, Lord, for whistling to me through the chaos of this life. I hear You.

Walking with Him

Listen closer. Think of a situation in your life that you have been praying about. Has the Lord answered you? Are you listening closely enough? Or are you selectively awaiting an answer that suits you? When you pray and listen closely for a reply, you will always hear the Lord—even when the answer runs contrary to what you want.

Fitness
Workout #8

Training at a Glance

Right about now you may be feeling that the warm-up isn't that necessary. Maybe you even feel silly jogging in place. Keep in mind, though, that although you're not necessarily breaking a sweat or feeling a lot going on as you warm up, the action is absolutely critical for your body before a bout of physical activity. Not doing it is like getting in your car every morning, turning it on and immediately flooring the gas. How long do you think you could do that before your trusty vehicle breaks down on you?

Before you begin the exercises, warm up by walking or jogging in place for three to five minutes. Your goal is to perform a total of at least one more rep than you did in your last workout on each exercise and in less total time.

Exercise	Reps Goal	Reps Rd. 1	Reps Rd. 2	Reps Total (2 Rounds)
Standard push-up				
Bodyweight squat				
Crunch				
Rd. time				

Firm Believer

The best way to utilize more oxygen and burn more total calories is to utilize whole-body movements. The more muscles working to perform an exercise, the better able you'll be to increase your at-work inner furnace as well as your resting metabolism.

Food Byte

Legumes like beans, peas and lentils contain healthy protein, fiber and carbs. Add them to salads, soups and grain dishes for a healthful, tasty boost. When you add a legume to a grain (such as adding beans to rice) you create a protein combo with all the amino acid building blocks that your body needs to recover and come back stronger.

Extreme Mind Makeover

Faith
The Exercise: Romans 12

To me, one of the most inspiring shows on television is *Extreme Makeover: Home Edition*. Each week, we get to take a look inside the personal hardship of a family and then watch as the team of architects, designers and construction workers completely transform their home. The living conditions that many of the families have endured, and the tremendous challenges they have faced due to a natural disaster, an illness or a disability touch your heart. What would normally take months to build, now takes only days.

But what's even more impressive is the transformation that God wants to bring about in our hearts and minds. His work is nothing short of miraculous. He literally does the impossible. My experience tells me that most of us are defeated in life by the way we think. Our "self talk" and thought patterns are predominantly negative, especially when we encounter challenges or obstacles or even plateaus.

Paul, who wrote the book of Romans, gets it. That's why he tells us that real transformation starts in our mind. God wants to tear down our old way of thinking. Paul knew that our thoughts would lead to beliefs, and that our beliefs would eventually affect our behavior. The reality is that if you do something over and over again, it eventually becomes who you are.

Listen to the way you think today—is it filled with optimism? Does it reinforce what God is capable of doing in your life? If you want God to transform your life, you have got to change the way you think.

—Page

Pastor's Point

1. What ways have you let negative thinking derail you from completing the things God has asked you to do?
2. Practice changing all of your defeated, discouraging thoughts into thoughts of faith and belief in what God is capable of doing.
3. Additional reading: Romans 12:1-2; Philippians 4:8-9.

Today's Prayer

Lord, help me to eliminate negative, defeated thinking. Help to me take every thought captive and use the truth of Your Word to change the way I think.

Walking with Him

The real goal of a changed way of thinking is life transformation. When our thinking improves—when we think on the things of God—our desires eventually come into alignment with God's best for our life. Then our attitudes and actions start to change as well. So, instead of focusing on how long it's been since you worked out, or how out of shape you are, insist on optimism and know that each day is an opportunity to be transformed into the likeness of Christ.

Fitness
Rest

Fitness in Focus: Progressive Overload. Simply put, you can't become fit without it. In the simplest of terms, progressive overload is simply the idea that in order to see continuous improvement and change, you must ask more of your body. I've said for years that the body will only change according to the level at which it is stressed. If you only do a certain amount of work or the same amount of work each day, you'll grow accustomed to it and you'll cease to improve.

Each day you attempt your workout, your goal is to do better in some form or fashion; either do more reps or complete your work in less time or tackle more exercises. And if it means just one more rep each day, that's fine. Remember, this isn't a sprint, but a lifelong commitment.

String enough reps together over the course of months and years, and you're sure to enjoy a healthier life.

As you continue each day, keep the idea of progressive overload in the back of your head. If you can do more than before, you know you're improving.

23,855

Number of deaths in the U.S. related to high blood pressure in 2006.

You Are Not Alone

Faith
The Exercise: 2 Kings 6:8-17

Mount Everest, the highest peak on earth, is undoubtedly one of the world's most difficult and dangerous mountains to climb. On the mountain, extreme temperatures, lack of oxygen, high winds and risk of avalanche can make this climb seem impossible. For even the most experienced mountaineer, the risk of death is always present. The truth is, it is virtually impossible to make the ascent to the summit without the help of the Sherpas. These guides make the ascent possible. If you were to try to go it alone, your chance of success would be virtually zero.

As a prophet of God, Elisha knew he needed help and that he was never alone. But as Elisha and his servant slept, the king of Aram sent horses and chariots and a strong force to confront them; they literally surrounded them and the entire city. The king was angry that Elisha always seemed to know their next move and was able to warn the Israelites of possible attack. Elisha's servant had woken up early only to see this vast army. Terrified, overwhelmed and isolated, he ran back inside to tell Elisha. But Elisha was unmoved. He was calm and confident. He didn't panic as his servant hid in fear.

Even though the situation looked impossible, he knew something that his servant didn't—they were not alone! Elisha told his servant to relax. He said, "Those who are with us are more than those who are with them" (2 Kings 6:16). Then Elisha prayed that God would open his servant's eyes to see a whole new reality—the spiritual realm where the battles are really won and lost. The servant's eyes were opened and for the first time he could see what Elisha saw all along—the hills were full of horses and chariots of fire. This was God's army.

Many times in life we feel alone. But we are never alone. In fact, not only are God's angels present, but His Spirit also lives in us to guide and teach and comfort.

Jesus never leaves us. On this journey of life, you are never alone.

—Page

Pastor's Point

1. Have you ever felt totally alone in life?
2. Do you find a calming presence during tumultuous or challenging times?
3. Additional reading: Psalm 91:10-12; Matthew 4:10-12.

Today's Prayer

Lord, thank You so much for always being there. Even when I'm facing the uncertainties of this life, You are by my side, laying a hand on my shoulder, calming my spirit. I pray, Lord, that I am always aware of Your presence— through rough seas or calm waters.

Walking with Him

Relax. Just like Elisha did. You find that people who are not walking with the Lord in this life tend to panic much more easily. When the economy takes a bad turn and drops their 401k into a 201k, they curse, weep and worry themselves into a frenzy when, really, all they need to do is look to the Lord. When the Lord is for you, who can really be against you? Faith. Obedience. Relationship. These are the things He asks of us. And know that even though you may not see it, those who are with us are more than those who are against us.

PrayFit Recipe of the Week
Feta Omelet with Tomato and Peppers

1 egg
3 egg whites
½ cup chopped tomato
¼ cup finely chopped bell pepper

1 oz. feta cheese, crumbled
Salt and pepper to taste
Nonstick cooking spray

Heat a nonstick skillet over medium heat. Combine egg and egg whites in a bowl, season with salt and pepper and whisk well. Add tomato and pepper to eggs. Spray skillet with nonstick spray and add egg mixture. Cook for 3 to 4 minutes until eggs begin to set; using a rubber spatula, gently pull in the sides of the omelet to let the uncooked egg run to the edges of the pan. Sprinkle feta over eggs and gently fold in half. Allow to cook for 2 minutes and transfer to a plate.

Calories: 223 | **Protein:** 22 grams | **Carbohydrates:** 8 grams | **Fat:** 11 grams

In 2010, heart disease will cost
the United States

$316.4 Billion.

This total includes the cost of
health care services, medications
and lost productivity.

An Eternal Warranty

Faith
The Exercise: Romans 5:6-9

"Well, your warranty is almost up, Mr. Peña," the service manager said when I took my pickup in to the dealership. My good and faithful truck seemed to be on its last rim when I sputtered and puttered onto the lot that day. But as he handed me the invoice, he said, "No charge! Ford will take care of the bill. But only for a little while longer."

"What was wrong with my truck?" I asked. But as he started down the list of valves and fluids that he replaced, my mind wandered back to what he said. My warranty was almost up. Soon it would be up to me to pay the debt. I found myself looking over his shoulder toward the new line of trucks on the lot.

"So, sign here. She's as good as new!"

Good as new? Well, I knew what he meant.

Later that night at the gym, as I stretched my aching back, I felt so thankful for my warranty. Not my truck's, but my own. Because not only can I get a daily inner tune-up from the Master mechanic, but someday I'll turn this old body in for a new one.

And when I stand before God's throne, with all my wear and tear, Jesus will say, "No charge. I have taken care of the bill. Forever."

—Peña

Pastor's Point

1. How "good" do you think you have to be to earn the Lord's eternal warranty?
2. How many times have you sinned and thought that the Lord would turn you away? Or that you had sinned one too many times for Him to welcome you back?
3. Additional reading: 1 John 1:9; Romans 10:9-10.

Today's Prayer

Lord, though I sport many imperfections, You have chosen to forgive me every time. Thank You for Your infinite grace. Help me keep my spirit in top working order on a daily basis.

Walking with Him

Service your soul. When we sin, we intuitively avoid the Lord. Like a child who would hide a broken dish from a parent, we choose to cover up the mistake rather than confront it. The Lord's warranty is the best in the business. Take your soul in for service each time you misstep, rather than waiting until sin further corrodes the engine.

Fitness
Workout #9, Baseline, Week 3

Training at a Glance

Have you found yourself sandbagging—if just a little bit—as you set your baseline for the week? You know, shave a little off of your initial workout session, so as to make your "one more rep" mantra a little easier in the upcoming workouts. If that sounds familiar, first forgive yourself, because it's human nature to want to set yourself up for success. But now turn that apprehension on its head and go all out by, well, going all out on this week's baseline. The rest of the week, put forth the intense effort needed to meet each day's goal.

Exercise	Reps Goal	Reps Rd. 1	Reps Rd. 2	Reps Rd. 3	Reps Total (3 Rounds)
Decline push-up*					
Bodyweight squat					
Lunge*					
Reverse crunch*					
Rd. time					

*New exercise

Before you begin the exercises, warm up by walking or jogging in place for three to five minutes. Your goal is to perform a total of at least one more rep than you did in your last workout on each exercise and in less total time.

New Exercises of the Week

Decline Push-Up
Focus: Upper chest, shoulders, back, abs

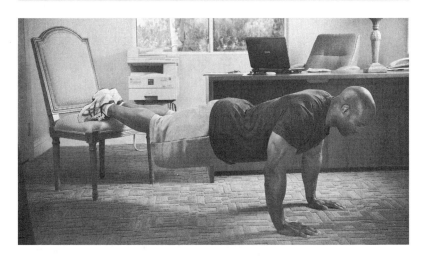

Get into a push-up position with your feet elevated on a stool, bench or couch. Place your hands wider than shoulder width apart and your eyes focused on the floor. Press yourself up to full arm extension, keeping your abs tight and back straight. Squeeze your arms and chest at the top, then lower yourself to the start. When your face reaches an inch or so away from the floor, explode back up to the fully extended position.

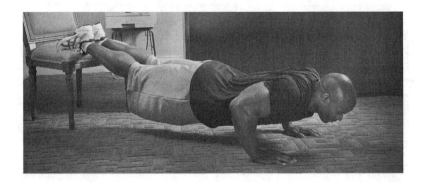

Reverse Crunch
Focus: Lower abs

Lie face-up on the ground with your hands extended at your sides, your feet up and knees bent at a 90-degree angle. Your thighs should be perpendicular to the floor. Slowly bring your knees toward your chest, lifting your hips and glutes off the ground, and try to maintain the bend in your knees throughout the movement. Return under control.

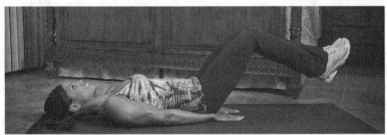

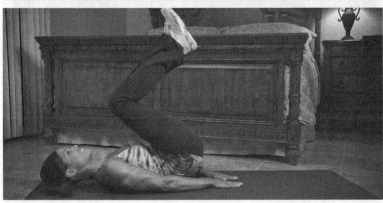

Lunge

Focus: Legs, glutes, hamstrings, lower back

Stand with your feet together, abs tight and eyes focused forward. Step forward with one foot. Bend both knees to lower yourself, making sure your front knee doesn't pass your toes on your front foot. Stop just short of your rear knee touching the floor and reverse directions, driving through the heel of your forward foot to return to the start. Alternate legs for reps.

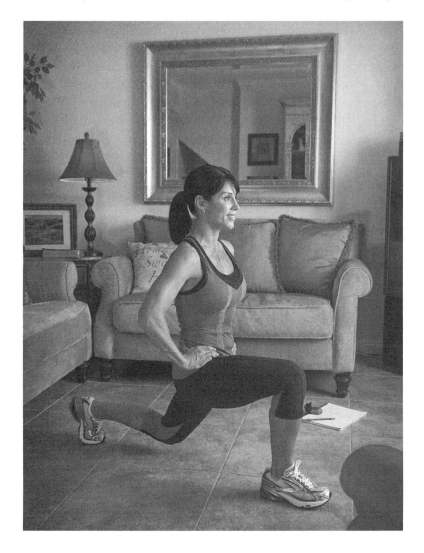

Firm Believer

Make sure you're journaling and watching the clock each workout in order to keep progression overload paramount.

Food Byte

Almonds are high in healthy monounsaturated fats and are an excellent source of vitamin E and calcium and protein.

Let Opportunity Knock

Faith
The Exercise: Joshua 1:9

There's one scene—well, make that one line—in the movie *Evan Almighty* that makes me pause. Allow me to set it up for you. God drops in on a congressman to help him change the world, since "changing the world" was the congressman's prayer. But when God asks him to build an ark in the middle of the desert, it becomes too much for his friends, co-workers and family to bear. And so here it is. God, dressed as a waiter, asks the wife, "Does God give us courage or does He give us an opportunity to be courageous?"

An opportunity to be courageous. How many times have we seen God allow things to happen in order for us to lean on Him? Let me explain.

Moses had Pharaoh; without Pharaoh, Moses would have had no one to set free. David had Goliath; better pick up a few mores stones for his brothers, because nobody was going to talk about God that way. And Daniel had his den. A new law was passed across the land that for 30 days, only the king could pray to God. If you prayed, you'd be punished. But Daniel would rather fall in the den than fall in line.

Moses, David, Daniel. Common men with uncommon courage, who saw obstacles as opportunities. I say we follow their lead. Are you facing an impossible dilemma? Make miracles with Moses. Problems at work too big to handle? Ask David for a stone. The crowd at school going in the wrong direction? Then turn and join Daniel in the den. When opportunities knock this week, seize them. It's God who allowed them in the first place. In fact, I've gotta go. There's someone at the door.

—Peña

Pastor's Point

1. When was the last time you acknowledged that God was using adversity as an opportunity in your life?
2. How did it turn out for you? For the others involved?
3. Additional reading: Deuteronomy 31:6-7; Luke 1:37.

Today's Prayer

Lord, I thank You for giving me opportunities to be courageous, because it forces me to depend not on my own strength, but on Yours. Help me to identify specific opportunities each day to rely on You.

Walking with Him

Nothing is too big for God. Often we believe that what we are facing is insurmountable; but with God, nothing is impossible. Take that first step of faith and watch how God shows up to save the day.

Fitness
Workout #10

Training at a Glance

You've mastered the incline push-up and the standard push-up. Now it's your opportunity to try the decline version, which (counterintuitively, based on the name) targets your upper pecs, often the weakest area of the chest. Enjoy the slightly different feeling it gives you in the working muscles.

Exercise	Reps Goal	Reps Rd. 1	Reps Rd. 2	Reps Rd. 3	Reps Total (3 Rounds)
Decline push-up					
Bodyweight squat					
Lunge					
Reverse crunch					
Rd. time					

Before you begin the exercises, warm up by walking or jogging in place for three to five minutes. Your goal is to perform a total of at least one

more rep than you did in your last workout on each exercise and in less total time.

Firm Believer

Since your goal for each exercise, each time through, is positive failure— the point where you can no longer properly perform any more reps of a given exercise—it's important to assess your limits. However, do not discount the ability of the body to do what is asked of it. Whenever my clients think they cannot possibly go on any further, I encourage them to do one or two more. And guess what? They deliver. You'll find that by encouraging your body to give you "one or two more," you can start to skyrocket your numbers very quickly.

Food Byte

Get an extra dose of omega-3 fats from flaxseeds and walnuts. These foods contain a different type of omega-3 than fish, so mix it up for all the healthy benefits.

Born Again

Faith
The Exercise: John 3:1-8

Can you imagine the scene? Nicodemus, the teacher of Israel, came privately to Jesus after the sun went down to ask Him deep spiritual questions. He had seen the miracles and knew that God was with Jesus. And I believe that deep down inside he longed for more of what Jesus had—the power, the peace and the intimate presence of God.

As a Pharisee, Nicodemus lived by the strictest possible religious rules. He was a man of high moral character, and he lived by the Book. By today's standards, he would be known as an upstanding member of the community and would probably have a spotless reputation. He was a good man, but he knew that he was missing something. He was attracted to Jesus because he knew that Jesus had what he was missing.

I don't believe that he came at night because he didn't want anyone to know. Instead, he didn't want to be interrupted by the foolishness and sneaky traps set by the rest of his Pharisee friends. He sincerely wanted to fill the void he felt in his soul. So when Jesus told him that in order to experience eternal life he had to be born again, Nicodemus was confused. How could that be? It was impossible to return to the womb and be born a second time.

But Nicodemus finally figured it out. All of his religious activity was meaningless because his spirit was dead. Believing in Jesus would finally bring him the life that he was seeking. No matter how good you think you are, you will never be satisfied until you have Jesus.

—Page

Pastor's Point

1. Have you ever felt like all of your "religious activity" didn't quite bring you what you thought it would?
2. How does Jesus link belief in Him with being born again (see John 3:15-16)?
3. Additional reading: Colossians 1:15-22; Philippians 2:8-11.

Today's Prayer

Lord, I am thankful for the gift that You have given me in Your Son, Jesus. Thank You that You have brought me back to life and made me part of Your family forever.

Walking with Him

Come to Jesus. Not just when it's convenient. Not just when it's quiet. Not just when you think no one is looking. Not just when you think you're expected to. The world would have you give in to all of the day's interruptions and clamor, making time for everything but Jesus. Today, practice checking in with Jesus often, whether in an understated prayer or a bold assertion before others.

Fitness
Rest

Fitness in Focus: Stretching. Let's talk a little about the idea of stretching as it relates to performance at home or in the gym: when you should stretch, what stretching is for and when stretching is ill-advised.

- **Don't stretch cold muscles.** By now many of you may have heard that you never want to stretch a cold muscle. Think of a muscle like a sponge. A sponge doesn't move all that well when it's dry, but soak it in water and it moves effortlessly. The same goes for our joints and muscles. Allow for water and blood to fill the areas and our bodies move with fluidity. That's why doing a proper warm-up is critical before you ever stretch a muscle.

- **Understand the purpose of stretching.** Flexibility in today's conversation is for range of motion purposes only. In other words, if you have the necessary range of motion in your arms, shoulders and chest to perform a push-up, you don't need to stretch your chest prior to the exercise. That's why we don't have you stretching each day of the workout. You can just warm up and go. In fact, the truth is, many people actually injure themselves because they overstretch prior to an exercise, yet they blame the injury on the exercise itself.

- **Get with the new school of stretch.** Research also confirms two things about stretching that you may not have realized. In sports competition, just as many people who stretch injure themselves as those who don't stretch. Also, if you stretch a muscle prior to an exercise, you'll be weaker at the site that was stretched. Now, again, we're not talking about functional flexibility (low back, neck, and so on) but rather the target muscles within a particular workout. If you have the necessary range of motion necessary to do the work, save the stretching for after your workout when you have a lot of water and blood at the target site and you don't care if you lose the natural tension in the muscle, which is key to performance. Done during this window, stretching can actually promote overall flexibility, kick-start recovery and help you fortify yourself against injury.

Time Can Wait

Faith
The Exercise: Isaiah 40:31

If there's one thing I demand of myself on a daily basis, personally or professionally, it's being on time. And I mean prompt! Whether it's a conference call, appointment or a meeting across town, I try to avoid being late, at all costs. Do I always come through? No. Are there times when I'm tardy? Absolutely. But being late bothers me to no end.

This morning, the world worked against me in this department, and I was running late. "Lord, help me get there on time," I'd mumble between grumbles. And just then I'd see daylight between cars, more brake lights, another stop. Just plain misery.

Well, I arrived to my appointment at the top of the hour. Rushing away from the truck, I got a message on my phone that my appointment was running 20 minutes behind. Despite my despair, even though I was late, I was early and therefore right on time.

Mary and Martha understood real despair in the area of being on time; Lazarus had already died. But was that the Lord approaching? Moses, as he was being chased by an angry pharaoh, was short on time and facing an angry sea. But was the Lord really parting the waters? And a group of scared disciples, grasping the edge of the boat, knew it was a matter of time before they sank. But was that Jesus in the water, strolling toward the boat?

What these biblical accounts have in common is not that time was of the essence, but rather, nothing good happened until God showed up. When God showed up, Lazarus walked out of the tomb; when God showed up, the Israelites walked on the floor of the Red Sea; and when Jesus showed up, Peter walked on water. First the waiting, then the walking.

Don't be mistaken: things didn't happen *just* in time or even right *on* time, but in *God's* time.

—Peña

Pastor's Point

1. Have you ever become discouraged with the Lord because something didn't happen when you wanted, hoped or expected?
2. What can you learn about waiting on the Lord's timing?
3. Additional reading: Romans 8:23; Psalm 40:1.

Today's Prayer

Lord, help me learn patience in all things. Give me the wisdom to see that when things don't happen according to my timetable, they are sure to happen according to Yours.

Walking with Him

Figure out why the Lord is making you wait. Praying for the Lord to bless you with a spouse, for example, might not be happening as fast as you'd like. Are there areas that the Lord wants you to grow in first? Does He just want you to trust Him and focus on other things? Ask Him.

Fitness
Workout #11

Training at a Glance

With the squat and lunge done back to back in this workout, you are really taxing your lower body. This is exactly the design—the muscles located there, from the gluteus maximus to the quadriceps to the hamstrings, are major movers and can take a lot of punishment before they respond by growing denser and stronger. Just don't let your concentration or form wane on the lunge due to fatigue: Stay focused and fight through it.

Before you begin the exercises, warm up by walking or jogging in place for three to five minutes. Your goal is to perform a total of at least one more rep than you did in your last workout on each exercise and in less total time

Exercise	Reps Goal	Reps Rd. 1	Reps Rd. 2	Reps Rd. 3	Reps Total (3 Rounds)
Decline push-up					
Bodyweight squat					
Lunge					
Reverse crunch					
Rd. time					

Firm Believer

Spread the word about what you've been doing. Keeping others informed about your routine will encourage you to keep with it.

Food Byte

What you drink is just as important as what you eat. Keep your fluid levels in check, especially when exercising. Carry a refillable water bottle with you at all times and drink throughout the day.

Tell Me About It

Faith
The Exercise: Philippians 1:3-6

Are you having a tough week? As I typed that sentence, I took a deep breath and sighed. Maybe you're doing the same as you read it.

Any missed opportunities on your mind? Some pitfalls you could have avoided? Any do-overs you'd like to have? I could think of a couple in my week.

But isn't it amazing, as much as it is encouraging, to know that we can curl up in the lap of God and tell Him all about it? (He knows our story. He wrote it but likes us to tell Him about it anyway.)

So make a list of things that stick out in your mind from this week—good, bad or ugly. Take a few minutes to think and pray about each one, giving thanks. The fact that I'm writing and you're reading is an awesome reminder that God is still working.

So go ahead, take a deep breath and sigh. Imagine God doing the same and saying, "Okay . . . tell me all about it."

—Peña

Pastor's Point

1. When you're having a tough week, who do you confide in?
2. Have you ever found yourself relying too much on another person, wondering if God is listening at all?
3. Additional reading: 1 Corinthians 1:8-9; Hebrews 11:6.

Today's Prayer

Lord, You are God, my Creator, my Savior. You are also my best friend. Though You know my troubles and triumphs, You still want me to share them with You, and I am all too happy to do so. Help me, Lord, to remember that no matter how many friends I have that I can seek the counsel of, it is Your reassurance and guidance that matter most.

Walking with Him

Converse with the Lord. Have an out-loud, de facto dialogue with Him. He does know our story, but He wants to hear it from us. Our faith is based on relationship. Our Sovereign Creator doesn't just rule from on high—He actually wants us to engage Him in conversation and seek Him with all our hearts.

Fitness
Workout #12

Training at a Glance

This week, you've traded the standard crunch, which targets your upper abdominal region, for the reverse crunch, which targets the muscles of the lower midsection. Did you notice a difference in how many reverse crunches you can do versus regular crunches? Don't worry—this is absolutely normal, as the lower abs traditionally lag in strength. Just do your reverse crunches slowly, do them correctly and do as many as you possibly can.

Exercise	Reps Goal	Reps Rd. 1	Reps Rd. 2	Reps Rd. 3	Reps Total (3 Rounds)
Decline push-up					
Bodyweight squat					
Lunge					
Reverse crunch					
Rd. time					

Before you begin the exercises, warm up by walking or jogging in place for three to five minutes. Your goal is to perform a total of at least one more rep than you did in your last workout on each exercise and in less total time.

Firm Believer

Recheck your diet. Have you been sticking to the meal plan outlined in this book or are you veering off the path a little? Your diet may be to blame for a sudden drop in energy levels.

Food Byte

Next time you fire up the grill for dinner, toss on some extra chicken breasts for quick and easy salads and sandwiches later in the week.

Identity Theft

Faith
The Exercise: Daniel 1:6-7

In today's culture, a name has very little importance. When we are choosing names for our kids, most of us just choose names that we like. We don't realize that every name has a meaning, or if we do, we are more concerned with how the name sounds or goes together with our last name.

In fact, most of us have become so casual with names that we allow our kids to address adults by their first name; and then we try to dress it up a bit by making them say "Mr. John" or "Mrs. Sue." But in ancient times, names had weight. And when the four Israelites were chosen for the king's service, their names had to be changed. After all, Daniel means "God is my judge"; Hananiah means "The Lord shows grace"; Mishael means "Who is what God is?"; and Azariah means "The Lord helps."

Nebuchadnezzar would never allow these names to remind him that he wasn't God. So in order to make their identity theft complete, he changed their names. But since these men were completely devoted to God, he couldn't change who they really were.

As a Christian, you have been given a new identity as well.

When you place your faith in Jesus, you have become a new creation. Those who have believed in His name have been given the right to be called His children. Your name has been changed—and the essence of who you are has been changed too. The old nature is gone and the new has been given.

You no longer live—it is Christ living through you.

—Page

Pastor's Point

1. As a Christian, how do you feel about the fact that your name is now His name?
2. Real identity change happens from the inside out. What areas of your life need to be changed?
3. Additional reading: John 1:12; Galatians 2:20.

Today's Prayer

Lord, I pray that I would live a life worthy of the name You have given me. I pray that You will change me from the inside out and that You will expose areas of my life that need to change.

Walking with Him

Pick an area of your life that you know needs change, and then change it. This very likely will not happen overnight; but by determining to change it, you likely will have taken more steps in the right direction than you ever have before. That's because tackling sin head-on, with the Lord at your side, is the only way to exact change. And remember, that "old you" is gone forever; the slate has been wiped clean. He will do remarkable things in your life.

Fitness
Rest

Fitness in Focus: Know Thy Abs. Even though you cannot completely isolate any one portion of the abdominals, you can involve to a greater extent a particular section over another through exercise selection. So, if you attack your abs with all sorts of moves, you're sure to cover the bases for a balanced midsection. And strong abdominals mean a well-protected low back.

- **Lower Abs.** The lower abs are the weakest link along the chain of ab muscles. The key to targeting the lower abs is to bring your legs toward your torso, as you do in reverse crunches and hanging leg raises. If your lower abs are a weakness, try doing them first in your ab routine and increase the frequency of these workouts throughout the month.

- **Upper Abs.** The most recognizable section of the abs are also the strongest: the upper abs. But it doesn't mean you don't need to concentrate on them. Any time you bring your torso toward your legs, you target the upper abs.

- **Obliques.** Helping complete the abdominal package are the internal and external obliques, which are responsible for trunk rotation and lateral flexion of the torso. Strong obliques are also integral to athletic performance, no matter the genre. If you've neglected your obliques, the imbalance will be detected immediately when you begin these exercises. A dedicated approach will help bring balance to your midsection.

- **Core.** While all of these muscles we've been working make up the overall core, here we're specifically talking about the innermost abdominal muscles. You can think of the transverse abdominis as an internal weight belt, helping provide stability to your spine by producing intra-abdominal pressure. This pressure, much like that provided by a weight belt, helps keep the spine in safe alignment during all the other exercises, protecting you from injury. A weak inner core is susceptible to the spine traveling forward toward the navel, causing injury.

Every year about

785,000

Americans have a first heart attack. Another

470,000

who have already had one or more heart attacks have another attack.

Put God's Ways to the Test

Faith
The Exercise: Daniel 1:9-20

I just love a good ol' fashion showdown. Like those old Westerns where the good guy squares off with the villain in a life-and-death quick draw. John Wayne was a master at this.

I get the impression that Daniel engaged in the same kind of situation when he asked the king's official to put them to the test. But the reality was this: Daniel was actually putting God on the spot. He knew that God's ways were best, and he didn't want to violate his convictions. So Daniel was willing to put everything on the line when he said he wanted to eat God's way.

Now Daniel probably didn't know for sure how everything was going to turn out, but he was willing to walk by faith and trust God for the result. I'm sure it would have been much easier to just go along with what everybody else was doing, especially since his entire life had been turned upside down. But Daniel decided to take a stand—again.

It is not easy to take a stand in the face of social pressure.

Doing things God's way means that we are choosing to take a different road than most. But we have a God that we can trust. We can be confident that His ways are best—that He will deliver us one way or another.

—Page

Pastor's Point

1. What are some areas in which you know you need to obey God, but you aren't sure how it will turn out?
2. What decisions can you make that will cause you to go against the flow?
3. Additional reading: Acts 20:22-24.

Today's Prayer

Lord, I pray that You give me the strength to go against the flow, even when everyone around me isn't. Help me to resist the influence from my peers.

Walking with Him

Accept the challenge. The thing is, of all the Lord's promises, He never assures us that life will be easy. In fact, it's quite the opposite. Being Christian assures you of persecution and trials. His promises surface on the other side of the challenges in this life. But you should never shrink in the face of social pressures. Today, identify and eliminate some of your conformist behaviors that might be keeping you from a deeper relationship with the Lord.

PrayFit Recipe of the Week
Simple Baked Salmon

5 oz. skinless wild salmon fillet
2 tsp olive oil
1 tsp chopped rosemary
Salt and pepper to taste
3 slices fresh lemon

Preheat oven to 375º F. Place salmon on a baking sheet lined with parchment paper or aluminum foil. Drizzle with olive oil and sprinkle with rosemary, salt and pepper. Top with lemon slices and bake for 15 minutes until just cooked through.

Calories: 287 | **Protein:** 31 grams | **Carbohydrates:** 0 grams | **Fat:** 17 grams

42% Higher
The medical costs for an obese person compared to someone of healthy weight.

Most Valuable Prayer

Faith
The Exercise: Philippians 3:14

Few things in sports are as exciting as the last-second shot. The buzzer beater or walk-off homer are what the games are all about. We've seen our share of miracles on ice to know that it ain't over till it's over. And we love to watch the highlights.

You know, that's one thing that sports teams do very well: they watch film. After each week's game, they play it back. They rewind and fast forward, analyzing each play to determine why something happened and how to make it better. Film can be both beautiful and brutal.

Of course, there's no film for us to watch on our week, but we all know inside our hearts if we ran the right routes. "Did I misread someone's cry for help? Did I miss an opportunity to stick up for someone? And, *ouch*, if I'd only avoided that conversation, I wouldn't have the regret of gossip."

The scoreboard of life would be unbearable if it weren't for the Lord, because despite our fumbles, missed grounders and air balls, He's there. He's the ref on the court, the coach on the field, and our Daddy in the stands. And best of all, He's already defeated our opponent.

As you enter this week, think ahead to your Friday highlight reel and take the shots that matter when the game is on the line.

—Peña

Pastor's Point

1. What does having an eternal perspective do to your earthly mindset?
2. How often do you look back at a week and see missed opportunities?
3. Additional reading: 1 Peter 3:15; Colossians 4:6.

Today's Prayer

Lord, there are so many ways that You can use me to show Your love in this world. Help me see those opportunities and do Your will in each instance.

Walking with Him

Be a pressure player. Over the course of the week—school, work and home—there are plenty of chances to demonstrate your faith, not just for yourself but also on behalf of others. Be bold this week, keeping your faith radar on high alert for opportunities to be a clutch performer for the Lord.

Fitness
Workout #13: Baseline, Week 4

Training at a Glance

Your training session has stretched to seven exercises, but there's nothing you haven't seen before. In fact, you know these moves now pretty well, so tackle them with confidence and wield them for what they are: tools to transform your health, your fitness and your very relationship with your body.

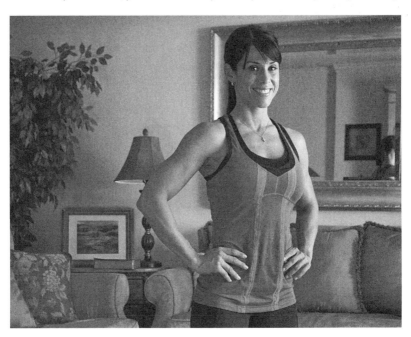

Exercise	Reps Goal	Reps Rd. 1	Reps Rd. 2	Reps Rd. 3	Reps Rd. 4	Reps Total (4 Rounds)
Decline push-up						
Standard push-up						
Incline push-up						
Bodyweight squat						
Lunge						
Crunch						
Reverse crunch						
Rd. time						

Before you begin the exercises, warm up by walking or jogging in place for three to five minutes.

Firm Believer

Get plenty of rest. You should be getting seven to nine hours of sleep in order to support the work you're doing on this program. Try to reduce the number of roadblocks standing between you and an earlier bedtime.

Food Byte

Getting tired of steamed or boiled veggies? Roasting at high heat brings out a sweet and nutty flavor that you can't get from steaming. Try roasting broccoli, squash, sweet potatoes and cauliflower—you won't believe the flavor boost.

The Recruit

Faith
The Exercise: Luke 5:5

Smelly, dirty, grimy—these are just a few of the ways to describe Peter and his buddies. After all, they spent their days baiting hooks and cleaning fish. I'm smiling as I picture Jesus the recruiter walking up to this crew. Did He pause and grin, crouching down to watch and listen to them work? Maybe after a few minutes He looked skyward with a smile as if to say, "I found them."

I'm not sure, but I like to wonder what happened in that moment just before the call. What we do know is that of all the fishermen that came off the water, this bunch caught God's attention. And not long after Christ borrowed Peter's boat, the two were catching fish in water too deep for the nets to reach—Peter's preview to the depths of His love.

So, as we start our cars, open our offices, enter our cubicles or prepare for housework, let's do what Peter did and abandon control. Let's just imagine Jesus saying with a grin, "I found them," and this is that moment just before the call.

—Peña

Pastor's Point

1. Why do you think the disciples that Jesus recruited were chosen for the job?
2. Were they smarter or more talented than the rest? Or were they just willing and obedient?
3. Have you ever used the phrase "Because I say so"? Have you gotten the behavior you wanted after saying that?

Today's Prayer

Lord, I know that You didn't choose the brightest and the best. But You did choose those who were willing to follow Your lead, to listen and obey. Help me to be one of those who hears Your voice and knows that You always know best.

Walking with Him

Stop working so hard to be good enough. Jesus calls those whose hearts are His—those who will listen to His voice and follow where He leads. Just pay attention to what He tells you, and He will do great things through you.

Fitness
Workout #14

Training at a Glance

Picture what occurs in your body as you do the incline, decline and regular push-up. See in your mind's eye your pectorals and triceps flexing to lift your body upward, and then elongating under tension as you lower yourself. Being aware of the actions of your various muscle groups helps you develop what's referred to as a mind/muscle connection. Developing that connection can help you consistently avoid the pitfalls of an unproductive, "going through the motions" session.

Exercise	Reps Goal	Reps Rd. 1	Reps Rd. 2	Reps Rd. 3	Reps Rd. 4	Reps Total (4 Rounds)
Decline push-up						
Standard push-up						
Incline push-up						
Bodyweight squat						
Lunge						
Crunch						
Reverse crunch						
Rd. time						

Before you begin the exercises, warm up by walking or jogging in place for three to five minutes. Your goal is to perform a total of at least one

more rep than you did in your last workout on each exercise and in less total time.

Firm Believer

While the *PrayFit* program doesn't offer any specific guidelines on cardio—the high-octane nature of these workouts provides plenty of heart-racing, fat-burning benefits—you are free to engage in other exercise if you (a) have energy to burn or (b) would like to augment your training. But temper your volume; in other words, don't finish a workout here, then head out for a 10-mile run. If you increase your workout frequency, intensity or volume too much, your body will start to work against you.

Food Byte

A study from the Scripps Clinic (San Diego, California) reported that subjects eating half of a grapefruit or 8 ounces of grapefruit juice three times a day while maintaining their normal diet lost an average of 4 pounds over 12 weeks. Researchers reported that the effect is likely due to grapefruit's ability to reduce insulin levels.

Train Right

Faith

The Exercise: 1 Corinthians 9

Famed football coach Vince Lombardi once said, "Winning isn't every-thing. It's the only thing."

I have never met an athlete who didn't want to win. Not one. But wanting to win and doing what is necessary to win are two different things. Even Paul, a non-athlete, knew that an athlete would have to train right in order to have an opportunity to win.

Paul knew that self-discipline, focus and proper training techniques would all be required to get the prize. We have access to information overload today—just take a quick walk through your local bookstore and you'll literally see hundreds of books with the newest approach to healthy living, nutrition and exercise. We have logs and blogs and even access to the experts, yet we continue to get bigger and unhealthier.

The same is true of our spiritual life. It's virtually impossible to grow into the likeness of Christ without a strict spiritual training program. But most of us don't approach our spiritual life with the focus and discipline required to get the prize that lasts forever. We're often lazy with respect to reading and knowing God's Word. We're undisciplined in our prayer time. And we find ourselves unprepared for the challenges of life.

Spiritual training comes primarily through the foundational four: (1) intimate prayer, (2) meditating on God's Word, (3) Scripture memoriza-tion, and (4) accountability. Prayer puts us in a position of humility, sur-render and awe. It helps us realize and communicate our need of God. Meditating on His Word gives light to our path and makes our steps sure. Committing verses to memory gives us truth to fight against the attacks of the enemy. And accountability helps us keep our commitments and stay on track.

It's time to train right. It's time to approach our spiritual training with the same focus and tenacity we apply to our physical training, knowing that the prize will last forever.

—Page

Pastor's Point

1. Do you follow a daily spiritual training program?
2. What are the most important things you can do to become more like Christ?
3. Additional reading: 1 Timothy 4:7-8; 1 Corinthians 9:24-27.

Today's Prayer

Lord, I pray that I will have the strength to follow a plan for spiritual training so that I can grow in godliness. Help me approach my spiritual training with as much discipline as I do the physical.

Walking with Him

Incorporate some structure. If you find it difficult to set aside time for the Lord each day, schedule a time or times—literally. Whether it's upon waking or when you get home from school, the time you set up should be inflexible. *PrayFit* is a great tool for building consistency.

Fitness
Rest

Fitness in Focus: Bodyweight and the Staircase Effect. As we've said, the *PrayFit* program is built upon the concept of overloading the body each week. We've loaded the program with compound exercises, which are exercises that involve more than one muscle group to perform the moves. Because of that, compound exercises are commonly known as multi-joint exercises.

Using compound exercises like the ones we've chosen allows you to utilize more muscle groups at one time, giving you the opportunity to burn more calories in one workout session while also helping you tighten and tone your entire musculature with greater speed and success.

Hitting your entire body with workouts multiple times per week incorporates what we like to call the staircase effect. What that means is that training the same muscle groups multiple times each week allows you to build upon the effect of the previous workout. If you wait too long between workouts, you're back to square one, almost as if you are starting over from the original point.

That's why consistency—whether in this program, your reading or anything else in life—is the key to making progress.

1 out of every 3

kids is at risk of diabetes and will not outlive their parents.

Direct Sonlight Required

Faith
The Exercise: Proverbs 27:19

I recently looked in the mirror and said to my wife, "Babe, I think I'm vitamin D deficient. I think I need more sun." Seriously. I looked pale as a ghost, and I realized that for a few days, I'd been at my desk writing for so many different people and publications that I hadn't seen the light of day. Not only did my skin have absolutely no color or radiance, but my energy was also extremely low. Although I was feeding it correctly and drinking plenty of fluids, I was just "off." And no amount of coffee or protein would help. I simply needed to spend more time in the sun, and I knew it.

Don't we often feel that way spiritually? I know that I do. Even though I'm spending time with the best people and singing all the right songs, there are times when I just know I'm off. A little dull in my heart. Spiritually pale, with a real need of the Son. Maybe you can relate. Are you feeling deficient? Then step out of the shade of routine and into the Son's light. The more we turn toward Him, the better we'll reflect Him.

Soak up His energy and bask in the warmth of His promises. Besides, if we're going to be the light to a dark world, it's important that we stay plugged in to the Source.

—Peña

Pastor's Point

1. Do you feel that your life reflects the Lord's light?
2. Have you been experiencing a lull in your spiritual vitality? If so, why?
3. Additional reading: Mark 1:35; 2 Corinthians 3:18.

Today's Prayer

Lord, I know that I simply need more time with You. I have let the business of life crowd my time, and I desire more of You. Help me do whatever I need to do so that I can stay connected to You and reflect Your glory.

Walking with Him

Get involved. One of the best ways to make sure your light doesn't fade is to make yourself accountable to others. Join a small group, host a Bible study or even go on a missions trip. But most importantly, get daily time with Him. When you live in the light, it's tougher to become God-deficient.

Fitness
Workout #15

Training at a Glance

One thing you can keep in mind to maintain proper form during the body-weight squat is the position of your hips throughout the movement. On the descent, your hips shift backward (like sitting in a chair). Doing this will help ensure that your knees stay back and don't shoot out beyond your toes, which throws off your biomechanics. On the ascent, your hips shift forward to help bring you to a standing position. Think about this hip movement with each rep.

Before you begin the exercises, warm up by walking or jogging in place for three to five minutes. Your goal is to perform a total of at least one more rep than you did in your last workout on each exercise and in less total time.

Exercise	Reps Goal	Reps Rd. 1	Reps Rd. 2	Reps Rd. 3	Reps Rd. 4	Reps Total (4 Rounds)
Decline push-up						
Standard push-up						
Incline push-up						
Bodyweight squat						
Lunge						
Crunch						
Reverse crunch						
Rd. time						

Firm Believer

Does your neck hurt? Then perhaps you're committing one of the top all-time crunch form errors. When you perform a crunch, you're working your abs. Yet so many people end up working their necks because of how they perform it—clasping their hands behind their heads and pulling upward. This not only removes the focus from your ab muscles, but it can also cause both chronic and acute neck pain. A better way (and the right way) is to gently place your fingertips at the sides of your head. If this is still difficult for you, keep your hands off of your head completely until you learn to feel it where you're supposed to feel it.

Food Byte

Nuts and seeds aren't only for the bird feeder. These plant-based sources of protein and healthy fat are a great addition to your diet. Try an almond butter sandwich or some cashew butter on apple slices. Add sunflower or pumpkin seeds to salads and trail mix.

I'm Right Here

Faith
The Exercise: 1 Timothy 6:12

From where I sit, I can see a beautiful picture of a mountaintop hero. Standing atop the peak, hands on his hips, we're to believe he's just reached the summit. You've probably seen it or at least something similar. Underneath it reads one of my all-time favorite quotes from Theodore Roosevelt:

> The credit belongs to those who are actually in the arena. Who strive valiantly. Who know the great enthusiasms, the great devotions and who spend themselves for a worthy cause. Who, at their best, know the triumph of the high achievement. And who, at worst, fail. Yet fail while daring greatly, so that their place will never be with those cold and timid souls, who knew neither victory, nor defeat.

Sound familiar? I'm sure it does. But do you know what Mr. Roosevelt was speaking of when he wrote it? It's widely agreed upon that he was tapping his favorite sport of boxing to help illustrate a principle. His message? Get in the ring of life and fight. It's easy to watch from the stands, but the real hero is he who decides to accept the next challenge, reaches deep inside himself and goes for it.

Call me sentimental, but isn't that the way we need to approach each day? Shouldn't we be walking into our work, our schools, churches, grocery stores and gyms with a *God-is-in-my-corner* attitude? I mean, we serve the Maker of all matter, the King of the Ages. And yet we're often timid, afraid of our own shadow. Forget about witnessing to strangers; we're too busy avoiding cracks in the pavement.

I say we glove up. And whether we're at play, work or otherwise, let's mix it up like believers should. We might get knocked around a little, but at least we're daring greatly. Friends, the reality is, with each passing day, we're one round closer to heaven. But the fight's in the middle of the ring. In fact, I don't know where else I'd rather be when we hear that final bell.

—Peña

Pastor's Point

1. How boldly do you live your faith around others?
2. What is holding you back?
3. Additional reading: 1 Corinthians 9:25-26; 1 Timothy 1:18-19.

Today's Prayer

Lord, I am so grateful for each day and regret any that pass without my making a bold statement on Your behalf. Help me to be a bold believer today.

Walking with Him

Talk about God today. Mention your faith in passing. Talk about your last trip to church. Discuss how you prayed about something. These not-so-subtle illustrations of faith might reach someone who is in need of the Savior you've already found.

Fitness
Workout #16

Training at a Glance

As we mentioned in the last workout with hips and the squat, the hips are also a key factor in reverse crunches. For this exercise, you are lifting your hips up off the floor by flexing your abs. It's not a large range of motion, but keep your mind on your hips and you may have better luck in mastering this valuable movement.

Before you begin the exercises, warm up by walking or jogging in place for three to five minutes. Your goal is to perform a total of at least one more rep than you did in your last workout on each exercise and in less total time.

Exercise	Reps Goal	Reps Rd. 1	Reps Rd. 2	Reps Rd. 3	Reps Rd. 4	Reps Total (4 Rounds)
Decline push-up						
Standard push-up						
Incline push-up						
Bodyweight squat						
Lunge						
Crunch						
Reverse crunch						
Rd. time						

Firm Believer

Don't buy into the hype behind dedicated core (abs, lower back, hips and glutes) training. Trainers who would place you on a balance board or exercise ball for everything are ignoring two important facts: First, you cannot build as much strength when using these wobbly implements, making strength and muscle gain much slower. Second, major multi-joint moves like push-ups and squats do recruit your core musculature to a great degree. Sprinkle in some dedicated ab training with your regularly scheduled *PrayFit* routines and you'll have a strong, toned core—no balance board required.

Food Byte

Embrace variety. By eating a variety of foods, you are exposing yourself to a wider spectrum of health benefits. Everyone has his or her favorite foods, but eating the same thing day after day increases your risk of missing out on nutrients that are not found in those foods. Try something new or exotic. As you would be bold and adventurous for the Lord, be so with your nutrition! As a general rule, the more colorful your foods the better for you (this does not include neon-colored sodas and candies). Bright red, yellow and orange foods are rich in beta-carotene, and dark green and purple foods are generally high in antioxidants, calcium and minerals.

You Will Suffer

Faith
The Exercise: Acts 20:22-24

I can still remember the start of practice for fall sports coming off of a lazy summer. The intensity of the workouts was often magnified by two-a-days where we would practice in the morning and afternoon to get us in shape for the season. If you didn't do much to stay in shape during the summer, you were definitely going to be punished by the training.

Words like "suffering," "pain" and "hardship" are generally not what we look forward to experiencing. When is the last time you heard someone pray for anything on that list? Have you ever thanked God for pain, hardship and suffering?

The truth is, most of us will do everything we can to avoid those things; we would much rather experience God's blessings and His favor and success in all that we do. But Paul not only experienced these things on a regular basis, he was even led into them by the Holy Spirit. I'm not sure that I would be eager to do something if God told me that prison was waiting for me. Would you?

In many ways, this passage just doesn't seem to fit into our image of God—led by the Holy Spirit into hardships? Facing prison? What about making me lie down in green pastures or leading me beside quiet waters?

The next time you are suffering through a grueling practice or training session, remember Paul. God led him into situational suffering to produce fruit for the kingdom of God that would be everlasting. Whatever trial you are facing, whatever difficulty in your way, let that suffering be the crucible that brings great strength and refinement to your character and great confidence in God.

Are you up for the challenge? Are you willing to go where God leads to testify of His grace—even if it means hard times?

—Page

Pastor's Point

1. Have you ever obeyed God and suffered for it?
2. Does this idea that God leads us into hardships stretch your picture of God?
3. Additional reading: 2 Timothy 1:8-10; 2:3-5.

Today's Prayer

Lord, I know that life is not always going to be easy. But as hard times come, please sustain me and help me remain true to You. I will follow You, no matter where You lead.

Walking with Him

Think about hardships. Look back on your life and identify times when you have experienced significant situational suffering. Where were you with the Lord then? Did you pray for Him to bring you through it? Or did you feel as if He had abandoned you? What came as a result of those tribulations? Did you grow from it? Did someone else learn something?

Fitness
Rest

Fitness in Focus: Damage Prevention. Don't let a social event sidetrack your gains. Knowing what to do before a celebration where you might indulge in a big meal can make a big difference in your overall progress.

1. **Exercise early.** Try to sneak in a power workout. This will create a caloric deficit and a great window for muscle repair. This way, most of the calories to come are used to your benefit.

2. **Fill up on fiber and protein.** Before the family meal, try filling up on high-fiber, calorie-friendly fruits and veggies and take in 20 to 40 grams of protein from a high-quality source like turkey breast or a whey protein shake. This will keep you full longer, helping you to avoid a second—or third—trip back to the dessert table.

3. **Hydrate.** Drinking water—lots of it—will help you get a head start on leveling out your sodium levels. This, along with high fiber, will make you feel full longer, helping you avoid overeating.

Mind Games

Faith
The Exercise: Romans 12:2

Yogi Berra once said, "Baseball is 90 percent mental and the other half is physical." While Yogi's math might be a little off, he is right on target with the importance of training the mind.

After completing the Civil War Century ride, a grueling 105-mile ride through the mountains of Maryland and Pennsylvania, I was reminded of how important both physical and mental preparation are. It was a perfect day for riding, and I felt great physically, but I had never ridden beyond 50 miles. Although I regularly ride the hills, I was not prepared for the long, steep, 8-mile climbs throughout the day.

At the 70-mile mark I started to cramp up, first in my calves. I began to "super hydrate" in an attempt to prevent the inevitable. At about that point in the ride, there was a "bail out" where we could take a shortcut back to the start/finish line but not complete the full 105 miles. But I was determined to press on and complete the ride.

At the 85-mile mark, I saw other riders on the side of the road, suffering from cramps and rubbing their legs so they would be able to finish the ride. My cramping started to get far worse with every climb, and I had to dig deep to continue. My calves and now my quads were cramping severely. I had been praying for miles, but now my prayers were audible. I kept asking God to protect me from injury and to be my strength and shield. I am certain that my mental dependence on God throughout the race overcame my physical difficulties. I had many opportunities to shut down, but I was able to press on and finish.

Our Creator knows the power of the mind more than anyone. He even goes so far as to say that if we want to be different, if we want to be exceptional, if we want to be able to follow Him even when life is as tough as it gets, it all begins in our mind.

—Page

Pastor's Point

1. When you feel like giving up, does God's Word of encouragement come to mind?
2. Have you experienced real transformation in the way you think?
3. Additional reading: James 1:6-8; 2 Corinthians 10:5.

Today's Prayer

Lord, I pray that You would renew the way that I think—removing negative, pessimistic and critical thoughts from my mind. Give me the mental toughness to overcome great adversity.

Walking with Him

Get tough. It goes beyond positive thinking. Train your faith every day to be strong in the face of all challenges—physical and spiritual.

PrayFit Recipe of the Week
Ginger Chicken and Broccoli

2 tsp canola oil
5 oz. chicken breast, diced
1 clove minced garlic
2 tsp minced fresh ginger root
2 cups broccoli florets
2 tsp honey
1 tbsp reduced sodium soy sauce
½ tsp hot chili sauce (such as Sriracha) (optional)

Heat oil in a large skillet or wok over medium-high heat; add chicken and cook for 1 to 2 minutes, tossing gently. Add garlic, ginger and broccoli—

continue to cook and toss for about 5 minutes until chicken is cooked and broccoli is crisp-tender. Add honey, soy sauce and chili sauce. Cook for an additional minute and then toss well and serve.

72,449

Number of deaths from the complications of diabetes in the U.S. in 2006. Diabetes was the sixth leading cause of death in the country that year.

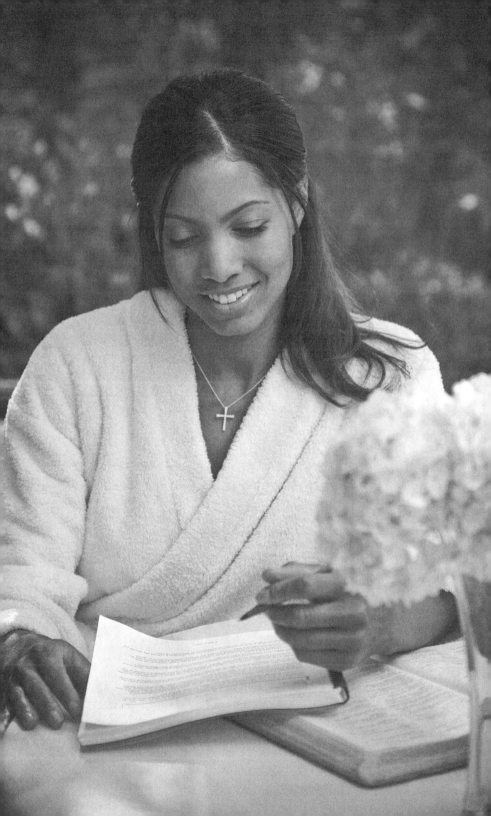

Month Two

Dig a Little Deeper:
28 Bonus Days to Help Keep You on Track

No matter the sport, vocation or job, there comes a time when it's tough to keep going.

You may be a fighter on the canvas; a soldier unsure of what lies beyond the hill; a mill worker on the night shift who hasn't seen his kids in days.

Different people, same struggle: putting one foot in front of the other.

And here you are. Do you have a fight on your hands? Are you in a battle? Is your family counting on you?

Then do what the best are able to do with God's help: put one foot in front of the other.

Welcome to Month Two. Carry on.

You don't have a soul. You are a soul. You have a body.

C. S. LEWIS

It's All About Who You Know

Faith
The Exercise: Ephesians 2:8-9

Recently, a buddy of mine asked me to join him at an exclusive black tie gala in Hollywood, celebrating some very accomplished people in show business (my friend being one of them). As we arrived at the host hotel, we were greeted with a hero's welcome. My door was opened for me, I was greeted by name, offered a beverage, escorted through the front door and given my all-access pass. Wow. An all-access pass. Boy, I felt important. My chest rose an inch and my confidence soared. Despite the fact that I did nothing to deserve the invitation, I was given freedom to go room to room with these VIPs. And in a surreal moment, as I sat there at dinner to celebrate the lives of these remarkable people, I realized, *I'm here, not because of who I am, but because of who I know.*

When I got home, I was cleaning out my pockets and found that all-access pass. I never did have to show it to anyone. I guess that was because everywhere I went my friend would say, "He's with me." And that was enough.

I can't help but think of another invitation that I'm glad I've accepted. Because someday, when I stand before the throne, and God looks upon my life, Jesus will say, "He's with me." And that'll be enough.

—Peña

Pastor's Point

1. Do you value earthly connections more than your connection with Jesus?
2. Do you feel proud to be associated with Jesus?
3. Additional reading: John 1:12-13; 3:15-17.

Today's Prayer

Lord, I thank You for inviting me to Your table. I am humbled by the fact that You think of me every day and that You desire to have me with You, even though I'm not always the perfect guest. Thank You for giving me an all-access pass to heaven and eternal life, not because I have earned it, but because I have believed in You and placed my life in Your hands.

Walking with Him

Check in with the Lord today. Realistically assess where you are in your walk with Him—are you walking beside Him, or have you paced yourself so far ahead of Him that you can't remember what it's like to feel Him near you? Be honest about where you stand with Him—you already know where He stands with you.

Fitness
Workout #1: Baseline, Week 1

Training at a Glance

It's Month 2, and we're guessing that, if you've stayed consistently on board the training program, you're feeling a heck of a lot stronger, more agile and more fit than you did a mere four weeks ago. Welcome to the transformative power of action! Knowing how far you've come, just imagine what the next 31 days or so will bring!

Exercise	Reps Goal	Reps Rd. 1	Reps Rd. 2	Reps Total (2 Rounds)
Plyo push-up*				
Bodyweight squat				
Crunch				
Reverse crunch				
Rd. time				

* New exercise

Before you begin the exercises, warm up by walking or jogging in place for three to five minutes.

New Exercise of the Week

Plyo Push-Up
Focus: Lower chest, shoulders, back, abs

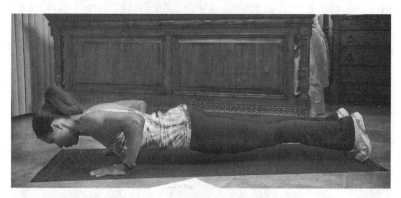

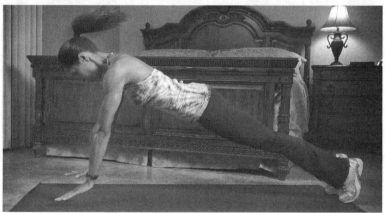

Get into a push-up position with your body in a straight line, feet to-gether, hands wider than shoulder width apart and your eyes focused on the floor. Explode yourself up to full arm extension, allowing your hands to leave the floor. Catch yourself with your hands on the floor, deceler-ate yourself to the start and repeat. Don't bounce your chest off the floor, but rather start each rep when your chest is an inch or so away from it.

Firm Believer
Time to build some power. Again, we're providing a fresh spin on the push-up. With the power push-up, you'll aim to generate enough power

through the ascent that your hands leave the floor on each rep. This works your overall pectoral complex but emphasizes your fast-twitch muscles, helping you build power and speed in this area. As with the standard push-up, it also places a heavy burden on your core as it works to maintain a rigid spine during each explosive rep. On the jump squat, you're working the same general principle. You will find that by combining these two into the same routine, you are left gasping for air—in a good way.

Food Byte

Speeding through meals is an American tradition that needs to stop. Eating too quickly can lead to stomach discomfort, excessive calorie intake and weight gain. Take your time, enjoy your food (and hopefully, some company) and you'll feel more satisfied.

Expires 1/1 of Never

Faith
The Exercise: Isaiah 40

There's been a big to-do lately about the validity of expiration dates on grocery store items. Without anyone regulating the shelf life of food, the business of labels is risky business. But no matter how soon we buy something or how well we preserve its freshness, time will eventually take its toll. Left to the elements, sooner or later we discover what's foul—and there's no mistaking when something's gone bad.

Truth be told, there's really nothing this life can offer that won't decay. Eventually, everything degrades, and thinking green won't be nearly enough to save the earth. Thankfully, God is imperishable, and we are not the world. He stamps a "BEST LIVED BY" on time itself. Not one thing about Him will ever get old or go bad. Not one promise, not mercy and not anyone He calls His own.

—Peña

Pastor's Point

1. God's Word is timeless and it reveals the character of God. How much time do you spend getting to know Him by reading His Word each day?
2. God's Word is always true. Do you look to the Word for answers to the important questions of life?

Today's Prayer

Lord, I am thankful that the truth found in the Bible is unchanging. I am thankful that You have given us answers to every question and that Your truth doesn't change with political correctness, the popularity polls or the changing culture. What's true is simply true. Thank You for giving me this sure foundation.

Walking with Him

Today, spend just 10 minutes reading John 1. Let His truth get into your mind and heart. Ask Him to apply His life principles to your day today. You can trust His Word for your life.

Fitness
Workout #2

Training at a Glance

Some of the world's greatest athletes play the most important games of their lives all the way through before they ever take the field. The idea of visualization—closing your eyes and imagining yourself successfully maneuvering through every moment of an upcoming activity, sport or event—is powerful. And you can do the same for your workouts to make them more productive. Before you begin, imagine how it will play out. See yourself breaking through your rep goals, and your body responding with grace and perfect form. It may take a few extra moments, sure, but the reward is better performance and a faster route to your goals.

Exercise	Reps Goal	Reps Rd. 1	Reps Rd. 2	Reps Total (2 Rounds)
Plyo push-up				
Bodyweight squat				
Crunch				
Reverse crunch				
Rd. time				

Before you begin the exercises, warm up by walking or jogging in place for three to five minutes. Your goal is to perform a total of at least one more rep than you did in your last workout on each exercise and in less total time.

Firm Believer

What's the best way to get in shape? The answer is simple: Find something you enjoy. These bodyweight exercises are a jump-start for you, but if you enjoy cycling, hit the road. Or maybe you have dreams of running a marathon. We could easily suggest cross-country skiing, but if it's not practical or something you enjoy, it's the worst piece of advice anyone can give. The more you enjoy an activity, the higher your chances of continuing that sport or exercise on a daily basis.

Food Byte

Take advantage of what the seasons have to offer—always choose seasonal fruits and vegetables when they are at their peak of freshness.

It's Just a Pebble

Faith
The Exercise: Judges 7

My wife recently took our youngest son out to lunch, and as they were leaving, my wife pushed against the door but it wouldn't budge. My son immediately came to the rescue and gave it his best shot, but once again the door barely moved.

They must have been making quite a bit of noise because another one of the guests got up and asked if he could help. And this guy was huge—the kind of guy who looked like a football player. My wife was sure the door was going to spring open. But the harder this man shook the door, the more obvious it became that the door was simply not going to open.

Thankfully, they were able to find an alternate exit and they left the restaurant. In their curiosity, they went back around to the other side of the door and immediately saw the problem—they found a tiny pebble about half the size of a marble that was caught in the door's threshold. My wife swept the pebble away and what do you know—the door swung open.

Sometimes the biggest obstacles in life are really just pebbles. But at the time, they seem insurmountable. When David faced Goliath, the challenge must have seemed insurmountable. When Gideon faced the Midianites with only 300 men, he must have felt the same way. But with God, our biggest obstacles become like pebbles. When we trust in Him and seek Him and give Him the glory, He shows us how small the obstacle really is.

—Page

1. How many times in life do pebbles stop us from opening doors?
2. Have you ever had a problem that seemed impossible to overcome?
3. How can you invite the power of God in to help you break through?

Today's Prayer

Lord, I pray that You would take my obstacles and expose them for the pebbles they really are. Help me to trust in Your power to overcome.

Walking with Him

Examine a problem you are currently facing. Could it be that the obstacle isn't as big as you think? Let God reveal to you the simple solution as you depend on Him to make things right.

Fitness
Rest

Fitness in Focus: Plyometrics. This month has introduced the concept of plyometric training. Plyometrics, or "plyos," are all about explosive power. When we were kids, we practiced plyometrics without even knowing it when we tried to jump as high as possible. What distinguishes plyos from other exercises is the element of acceleration; with plyometrics you don't slow down.

Take, for example, the squat jump exercise. For the first month of the program, you did bodyweight squats by bending at the knees and hips, lowering yourself to the floor, then standing up. With plyometrics, when you press yourself up, you explode upward off the floor. But you don't decelerate the squat jump—rather, you accelerate the movement to allow your feet to leave the floor. This concept of explosive training forces your body to trigger fast-twitch muscle fibers. That's an enormous benefit because it's the fast-twitch muscle fiber that has the greatest potential for increased tone and strength. And remember, the more muscle you possess, the more calories you will burn at rest. This metabolic kick-start helps you to make over your entire body composition faster than you would with lower-intensity exercise.

16

Percent of adults, 20 and older, in the U.S., from 2003 to 2006, who had high cholesterol levels.

The Gravity of It All

Faith
The Exercise: Proverbs 27

As if astronauts don't have enough to worry about, right? They've got the earth in the window while traveling at mind-bending speeds in frigid darkness, and, oh yeah—they're losing muscle mass and bone density by the second. It's a well-documented fact that they arrive back to earth drastically weaker than when they left. In fact, after only 11 days in space, they can expect to have lost as much as 30 percent of their muscle mass. Without the gentle, unnoticed tug of gravity, the body begins to wither away. The longer the time in weightlessness, the more painful and lengthy adjustment they go through when they finally get home.

We have a similar tug to keep us strong, don't we? The Holy Spirit whispers to our hearts and guides our steps, and we have friends and accountability partners to lean on us, encourage us and challenge us to keep our feet grounded in truth.

Thank the Lord for those who help form the gravity of our souls.

—Peña

Pastor's Point

1. Are you isolated from others who could be challenging you to grow spiritually?
2. Are you losing spiritual muscle because you aren't engaging with God or others about spiritual matters?
3. Faith needs to be exercised in order to grow. What area of your life do you need to hand over to God and trust Him with?

Today's Prayer

Lord, I don't want my faith to wither away. I desire to live by faith and trust in You. Please bring another believer along who will challenge me to grow and live for Christ.

Walking with Him

Write down a couple names of people who are strong in their faith. Invite them for coffee and ask them to push you to grow spiritually. We need each other to grow.

Fitness
Workout #3

Training at a Glance

Stop for a moment to reflect on your accomplishments. You've made it into the fifth week of the program. So many people who begin exercising quit on themselves, often before they even get this far, because they don't give their bodies a chance to respond. (It's estimated that 70 percent of people who begin a program drop out within six months.) But it's likely that you're already feeling a difference in your energy, stamina and strength—trust us, as working out becomes a natural part of your daily existence you'll start to feel like a day without training is incomplete, and you'll wonder how you ever did without it. That may be the best-kept secret of exercising: Once you're over the initial hump, you'll go from wondering how you'll ever keep it up to how you could ever imagine stopping!

Exercise	Reps Goal	Reps Rd. 1	Reps Rd. 2	Reps Total (2 Rounds)
Plyo push-up				
Bodyweight squat				
Crunch				
Reverse crunch				
Rd. time				

Before you begin the exercises, warm up by walking or jogging in place for three to five minutes. Your goal is to perform a total of at least one

more rep than you did in your last workout on each exercise and in less total time.

Firm Believer

Make things a competition. Whether it's simply against friends, your spouse or yesterday's best effort, always compete. Competition will help you continuously improve physically, and that translates to mental and intellectual progress as well.

Food Byte

When ordering or dining out, use these five tips to stay on track: (1) Check out the menu ahead of time to avoid a high-calorie impulse order; (2) Avoid creamy dressings, sauces and fried foods; (3) Have an appetizer portion as your entrée or split something with a friend; (4) Pass on the extra calories from breads and alcohol; and (5) Don't be shy—ask for exactly what you want and how you want it prepared.

God's Most Common Command

Faith

The Exercise: 1 Thessalonians 5

Of all the things God calls us to do, what does He require more than any other? No doubt it's to give to the poor. No, wait, I know—it's to love one another, for sure. What could be more important than that? Well, believe it or not, the most common command found in Scripture is to pray.

Without question, God wants to hear from us, from the times we need Him to when He deserves our praise. And since we've never lived one second when either reason wasn't true, I suppose we have our answer.

You know, it dawns on me we spend so much time on the phone, on Twitter or updating our status on Facebook when all the while God, our best friend, who loves us more than anyone, is hanging on our every thought. Like a proud new dad when he hears his child's first words, God is at the edge of His seat, ready to hear more. Can't you just see Him asking, "What's happening now?"

—Peña

Pastor's Point

1. Jesus modeled for us a life of prayer. He got away early to connect with His Father before the rush of the day.
2. Read Matthew 6:9-15. How does Jesus tell us to pray?

Today's Prayer

Lord, give me a desire to talk with You every day—to get quiet, to listen and to praise. Thank You that we can talk all day. And thank You that Your line is never busy.

Walking with Him

Consider adding the Lord's Prayer to the start and end of each day. Praise Him, ask Him to forgive your sins, thank Him for His provision and protection and ask Him to direct your path.

Fitness
Workout #4

Training at a Glance

Today, focus on your transitions. Are you wasting precious time or energy between your exercises? It can't hurt to see if you can be more fluid as you finish your push-ups and move on to squats, and then from squats to crunches. Think of yourself as a machine and seek out the most economical, efficient way to perform the workout, from beginning to end.

Exercise	Reps Goal	Reps Rd. 1	Reps Rd. 2	Reps Total (2 Rounds)
Plyo push-up				
Bodyweight squat				
Crunch				
Reverse crunch				
Rd. time				

Before you begin the exercises, warm up by walking or jogging in place for three to five minutes. Your goal is to perform a total of at least one more rep than you did in your last workout on each exercise and in less total time.

Firm Believer

Find a workout partner or use the *PrayFit* journal online. A trusted partner can serve as an accountability buddy and a source of healthy competition on a daily basis. Your chances of continuous progress increase dramatically if you're depending on someone, and vice versa. And if he or she is better than you, it'll help you reach heights you might not have reached otherwise.

Food Byte

Quinoa (pronounced "keen-wah") has whole grain goodness and more protein than any other grain. Add it to your pantry as an alternative to brown rice.

Are You an Elephant?

Faith
The Exercise: Philippians 4

Elephants are some of the biggest, most powerful and intelligent animals on the planet.

And in certain parts of Asia, farmers still use elephants to do much of the heavy labor. Some countries even hold elephant festivals to celebrate their strength and intelligence. These festivals always end with a tug-of-war between one elephant and 100 men—and you guessed it, the elephant always wins.

But think about this: The only thing that elephant owners in Asia have to do to control an elephant is tie a rope to its right hind leg and a small wooden post in the ground. That's it! And the elephant won't move, even though the wooden post and rope is no more significant than a toothpick and dental floss would be to you and me.

We can be a lot like those elephants. We have great strength inside us, but we struggle to remove the invisible barriers and limitations in our minds. We let doubts or fears and negative, destructive thinking keep us from reaching our full potential in our relationships, with our health and in all aspects of life.

Real transformation comes through the renewing of our mind. We have to change the way we think and refocus on godly things.

Isn't it time to break free from destructive thinking? Don't be like the elephant controlled by imaginary limitations.

—Page

Pastor's Point

1. In what ways do you think negatively or let doubts and fears hurt your performance?
2. List three things you can do to change your thought patterns.
3. Additional reading: Romans 12:2; 2 Corinthians 10:4-6; Genesis 6:4-6.

Today's Prayer

Lord, I pray that I will not be controlled by imaginary limitations. I depend on the power of the Holy Spirit to overcome my doubts and fears.

Walking with Him

Listen to your thoughts and words today. Make two columns on a piece of paper and write the negative thoughts on one side and the positive thoughts on the other. Which list is longer? Are there any patterns of thought that need to change?

Fitness
Rest

Fitness in Focus: The Upside of Failure. The *PrayFit* program is all about muscle failure. But what exactly is muscle failure? Muscle failure is the point during an exercise at which the muscles have fully fatigued and can no longer complete an additional rep of that exercise using proper form.

Now, in the gym world, research has indicated that taking every single set to failure is not recommended when using heavy weights; only your last few sets of each exercise should be taken to failure. Add to that the fact that when using heavy weights, you must wait days before training that muscle again.

But with the *PrayFit* program, we've not only built in ample rest days each week to ensure proper recovery, but we're also using bodyweight only (and by "only" we're not implying "easy"). By doing this, you're

safe to take each set to the point at which you can do no more, even from
the very first round of reps.

So, with *PrayFit,* there is no need to be afraid of failure.

9.1

**Percent of all medical spending
linked to obesity, up from 6.5
percent in 1998.**

Follow Me

Faith
The Exercise: John 10:10-30

I don't know about you, but I'm not too happy to be compared to a sheep. I mean, even though they're relatively clean, they still smell like an animal, they need somebody to constantly protect them, they're not very good with directions and they're not exactly the sharpest knife in the drawer. In fact, some would say they're just plain dumb.

But the good news about sheep is that they know the voice of their shepherd. They get to know that voice well.

When I was growing up, all the neighborhood kids would get together after school and then again after dinner to play games and hang out. But once it got dark, we knew we'd soon be hearing the voice of our parents, one by one, calling us home. Many times we couldn't hear our name, but we always knew which parent was calling.

As a dad, my kids know my voice. In fact, even in a crowded, noisy room, they're able to pick out my voice over all the others. And when I call for them, they follow. They follow because they know I love them, take care of them and they probably can't get home without me!

What a great picture of our relationship with Jesus—the Good Shepherd. When we spend time with Him by reading the Bible and praying, we get to know who He really is; it becomes easy to hear His voice and follow Him. And the best news is this—the path that He takes leads to eternal life. Can you hear His voice?

—Page

Pastor's Point

1. Why do we, like the sheep, need a Shepherd?
2. What are some ways that we can listen to Jesus and follow in His steps (see John 10:16,27)?

Today's Prayer

Lord, I pray that I would do whatever I need to do to hear Your voice clearly, follow in Your ways and experience Your presence and power.

Walking with Him

Let's be honest. Many of us don't spend enough time with Jesus to know Him. We can't recognize His voice because He is a stranger to us. Then we go to Him when we are desperate for help. Start to spend time with Him now so you will hear His voice clearly.

PrayFit Recipe of the Week
Turkey and Cheddar Panini

2 slices Ezekiel bread
2 tsp Dijon mustard
4 oz. deli turkey
2 slices tomato
¼ cup baby spinach leaves
1 slice low-fat cheddar cheese
1 tsp canola oil

Spread each slice of bread with mustard and assemble panini by layering turkey, tomato, spinach and cheese between slices of bread. Heat canola oil in a nonstick skillet over medium-low heat. Add panini and cook for 3 to 4 minutes per side, pressing down gently with a spatula. Cook until bread is toasted and cheese is melted.

Calories: 390 | **Protein:** 30 grams | **Carbohydrates:** 38 grams | **Fat:** 12 gram

220,000
Number of Americans who undergo gastro bypass surgery in the U.S. annually.

Trade Up

Faith
The Exercise: Job 13

The treelike features growing from his hands and feet were so gruesome, he'd become a national attraction. With barklike skin covering 90 percent of his body, his hands and feet were undetectable. This frail, now-35-year-old Indonesian known as Tree Man, was suffering from a wart-like disease he'd developed at 21, the likes of which doctors had never seen. The bark-like warts that covered every inch of his body would re-grow within days of being removed.

Quarantined for months at a time, Dede and his doctors got a call from an American physician who urged them to postpone any more surgery until they tried to treat Dede with injections of chemotherapy and Vitamin A. It was the American doctor's opinion that because Dede's immune system was so weak, unless they treated the disease from the inside, the warts would always reappear.

You know, being changed from the inside is how our Lord does His work. The gentle Shepherd holds us close. He sees the source of the problem—our hearts—and offers eternity's antidote. We might not have sores from head to toe, but without Him, we are terminal—carriers of a deadly illness with a specific cure.

And as for Tree Man? Well, doctors say he has years of rehab ahead of him, but the medicine worked. He got up and walked out of that hospital, having exchanged his hell for scars.

Have you exchanged yours for His?

—Peña

Pastor's Point

1. What we see on the outside always reveals something happening on the inside.
2. What in your internal environment needs to change?

Today's Prayer

Lord, I know that my words, attitudes and actions all come from what's in my heart. Only You have the cure for that. Please change me from the inside out.

Walking with Him

Stop trying to change your behavior. Let God reveal to you what's really going on in your heart. Ask Him to show you the source of your frustration or anger or jealousy. He will reveal it to you and apply just the right cure.

Fitness
Workout #5: Baseline, Week 1

Training at a Glance

Plyo push-ups followed by standard push-ups? Are we serious? In fact, we are. You may feel spent after a solid set of plyo push-ups, but you should still have a bit more power in your body to pump out some standard push-ups, as they require a bit less energy to complete. Embrace the challenge, and find the will to prove to yourself that you have what it takes to go the distance and beyond.

Exercise	Reps Goal	Reps Rd. 1	Reps Rd. 2	Reps Total (2 Rounds)
Plyo push-up				
Standard push-up				
Jump squat*				
Crunch				
Reverse crunch				
Rd. time				

* New exercise

Before you begin the exercises, warm up by walking or jogging in place for three to five minutes.

New Exercise of the Week

Jump Squat
Focus: Legs, glutes, hamstrings, lower back, calves

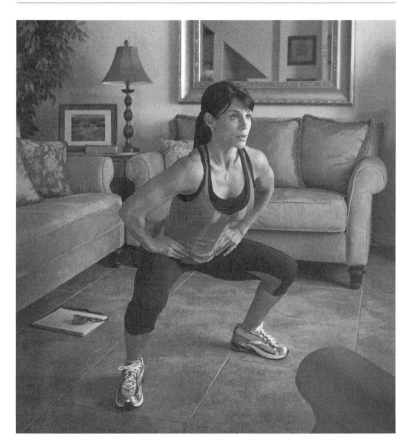

Stand with both hands directly in front of you, knees slightly bent and feet roughly shoulder width apart. Keeping your chest up and back flat, squat down until your thighs approach parallel with the floor, then explode upward as high as possible, allowing your feet to leave the floor. Land on soft feet with your knees bent and repeat immediately.

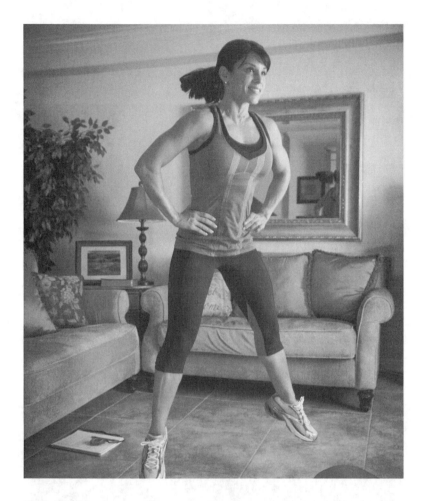

Firm Believer

The body will only change according to the level at which it is stressed; so that means doing more work each week. This is called the overload principle and is the bedrock of any and all successful programs.

Food Byte

Even though they are calorie free, artificially sweetened drinks can hinder your fat-loss progress. Drinking diet beverages can mess with your brain's ability to regulate calorie intake, causing you to feel hungrier. It can also cause you to rationalize taking in additional calories elsewhere.

Cooperstown

Faith
The Exercise: Ephesians 2

Virtually every sport has its version of a hall of fame—a place where the best players in history are honored alongside worthy peers. Arguably the most famous hall sits in a small town in New York. Get enough hits, runs and walks with few errors, and you just might get your name on the ballot and honored with enough votes for a trip to Cooperstown.

Well, in the lives of believers, heaven is the ultimate prize, where we'll walk the streets of gold alongside Paul, John and Peter. But it won't be because we batted 1.000 on earth. No, unlike Cooperstown, good earthly stats are sought not to earn heaven, but because of it. And when our names are read from the book of life, it won't be because of what we've done, but because of who we know.

—Peña

Pastor's Point

1. In what ways are you seeking the "praise of men" from your performance?
2. Examine your motives. Are you trying to earn God's favor? Are you trying to take some of the spotlight?

Today's Prayer

Lord, help me to live in such a way that I make Your name famous. I want my life to reflect Your glory. Don't let me take any of the glory that is rightfully Yours.

Walking with Him

In what ways are you seeking the praise of men? Are you trying to earn God's favor? Rest assured there is nothing you can do to earn heaven . . . nothing. It's a free gift of grace.

Fitness
Workout #6

Training at a Glance

When you do your jump squats, reach for the sky—literally. By bringing your arms back on the descent and swinging them forward on the leap, you can get more air. The higher you get, the more your muscle groups are not only working together, but working, period.

Exercise	Reps Goal	Reps Rd. 1	Reps Rd. 2	Reps Total (2 Rounds)
Plyo push-up				
Standard push-up				
Jump squat				
Crunch				
Reverse crunch				
Rd. time				

Before you begin the exercises, warm up by walking or jogging in place for three to five minutes. Your goal is to perform a total of at least one more rep than you did in your last workout on each exercise and in less total time.

Firm Believer

Always train abs last. You'll notice that we always ask you to work your abs and core last. The reason is, you want your abs and core to be as fresh and as strong as possible throughout an activity, since it's the core that supports your entire body and most importantly protects your spine. That's why the safest time to train abs is after everything else is exhausted.

Food Byte

Need a quick protein-packed snack? Crack open a hardboiled egg. They are quick, delicious and come in their own sterile package. Plus, you can prepare them in bulk at the start of the week so that you always have some on hand.

Invisible Fences

Faith
The Exercise: 1 Corinthians 10

I've got to tell you—I am so thankful for invisible fencing.

Every time I ride my bike I come across a ton of barking dogs. And a lot of times they really startle me, because I get in the zone as I ride and the barking is often a rude intrusion into my mental solitude.

Every time I see those dogs tearing after me, I hope and pray that they are either on a leash or contained by invisible fencing. If not, I don't think I would fare too well with my bike shoes, helmet and spandex bike shorts.

So I got to thinking that this situation is a lot like temptation in our lives. We often can see the temptation coming—and even though we aren't trying to find trouble, sometimes life, or even the enemy, just brings it our way.

But the great news is this: Even though temptation will come, we have the power to overcome it. God always provides a way of escape.

—Page

Pastor's Point

1. What are some situations you are currently facing that tempt you to do the wrong thing?
2. Can you clearly see the right path to take to avoid it, the path that leads to escape?
3. Additional reading: 2 Peter 2:4-9; 1 Corinthians 1:8-9.

Today's Prayer

Lord, I realize that all temptations have limits and that You always provide a way of escape. Help me recognize temptations early so that I can over-come. Thank You for protecting me from things I can't see.

Walking with Him

Sometimes we head into situations or relationships that we have no business pursuing. Are you currently engaged in tempting situations that have caused you to stumble? Maybe it's time to find your way of escape.

Fitness
Rest

Fitness in Focus: Muscle Soreness. You may have heard people say from time to time that they're sore and they need to get rid of the lactic acid inside their muscles. Well, to set the record straight, the accumulation of lactic acid that occurs during exercise has very little, if anything, to do with soreness in the hours and days following a rigorous training session or workout. The burn you feel from these push-ups, sit-ups and squats during the workout has a lot to do with lactic acid buildup, since lactic acid is a byproduct (waste product) and an indication of what's happening down inside our muscle fibers. But in truth, the lactic acid is long gone and flushed away within minutes and hours after the workout.

What's actually causing your soreness is literally microscopic muscle tears deep within. And because soreness usually takes a while to set in, scientists call it a delayed response, or delayed onset muscle soreness (DOMS).

DOMS, which sets in 24 to 48 hours after a tough workout and can peak up to 72 hours later, is that lingering stiffness you feel in the muscles you worked. In your case, you're probably feeling some discomfort in your chest, shoulders, legs, abs and glutes. While there is no way around DOMS, particularly at the start of a new fitness program, there are a few ways to help ease the pain.

1. **Walk it off.** Seriously. Taking a short walk—or a jog, if you can stand it—can help to circulate blood through stiff, stagnant muscles, helping to loosen them up. Afterwards, take advantage of the elevated blood flow by stretching. You can get similar effects by sitting in a sauna or hot tub, or simply taking a hot shower.

2. **Rest.** Resting a severely sore muscle or group of muscles is the best way to handle your soreness. Soreness, remember, is an indicator of actual damage, or tears, in the muscle, and resting to allow them to repair is key to your sustained progress and fitness.

3. **NSAIDs.** Nonsteroidal anti-inflammatory drugs (NSAIDs) are the pharmaceutical name for your favorite pain relievers like ibuprofen or naproxen. Taken as directed, these products can help relieve some of the hurt.

43

Percent of all Americans who will be obese by the year 2018; nearly 150 million people.

The Pain Principle

Faith
The Exercise: James 1

I am often asked what it takes for most people to actually make changes in their life, and I think the answer might surprise you.

I have found that there is one primary driver of change, and that driver is pain. Most people simply will not change until the pain of where they are is greater than the pain of making changes.

Whether it's financial pain, emotional pain or physical pain, we tend to make changes only when we're hurting. Unfortunately, pain is often the only thing that will get our attention to do the right things.

In Hebrews 12, God says that He even brings pain to get our attention when we have turned away from Him. And James 1 tells us that trials can have great purpose in our lives if we will just see them as God's way of refining our character and expanding our faith. When the bills are piling up and we are weighed down by debt, we will start to cut expenses. When our spouse threatens to leave, it wakes us up to start working on the marriage.

And every year millions of people start to eat right and exercise because they were just diagnosed with diabetes or had a heart attack or their doctor said they had to.

You have already made great changes to the way you do life. Stay on course. Don't fall back and return to your old ways. And remember that every challenge is simply an opportunity to get better and grow closer to God.

—Page

Pastor's Point

1. Is there sin in your life that is weighing you down? If so, what is it?
2. Can you see the ways that sin is hurting you as you walk with Christ?
3. Are you willing to confess those sins and be set free?
4. Additional reading: Hebrews 12:4-13; Proverbs 13:24; 1 Corinthians 11:32.

Today's Prayer

Lord, I pray that I will receive the trials in my life and see them as op-
portunities to grow in faith, perseverance and character. I know that
You only discipline those who You love.

Walking with Him

It's time to make changes before the pain comes. Don't wait for a trial to expose something that needs to change. Ask God what you need to work on, and go after it.

Fitness
Workout #7

Training at a Glance

During the push-up, which is mainly (and rightly) thought of as a chest, shoulder and triceps exercise, you may not necessarily real-ize it, but your back muscles are hard at work too. Be cognizant of the flexing of your latissimus dorsi muscles along each side of your outer back as you raise yourself up and lower yourself down. By be-ing aware of their action, you help forge a stronger mind-muscle con-nection, which leads to better form and more benefits over time.

Before you begin the exercises, warm up by walking or jogging in place for three to five minutes. Your goal is to perform a total of at least one more rep than you did in your last workout on each exercise and in less total time.

Exercise	Reps Goal	Reps Rd. 1	Reps Rd. 2	Reps Total (2 Rounds)
Plyo push-up				
Standard push-up				
Jump squat				
Crunch				
Reverse crunch				
Rd. time				

Firm Believer

The explosive movements in these workouts, such as the jump squat and power push-up, have an interval-like quality, and that's key. Intervals have you exercise at a high intensity for short periods, rest for another short period, then begin the exercise again. There's no exact set structure to intervals, but research has shown that you not only burn a higher percentage of fat per bout of exercise with intervals, but you also can actually preserve more muscle tone as compared to longer cardio sessions.

Food Byte

Wash and chop your salad greens and vegetables when you get them home from the store. Dry well and store in plastic bags in the fridge so they will be ready when you are.

Broken

Faith
The Exercise: Luke 22

Have you ever stopped to think about all the great and odd ways that God gets the attention of His people? Lazarus woke up, Jonah saw the inside of a whale and Peter heard a rooster. Just run through the Bible and you can find countless examples of jaw-dropping, head-swiveling surrender to God's presence and authority.

Although you and I don't cheat tombs or choke whales, we can all identify with Peter at the fire pit. How many opportunities to witness for Jesus have we allowed to go up in smoke—perhaps around the fire pit of jobs, school or the gym? Like Peter, we all know how it feels to disappoint Christ; and though we would like to turn back time, Christ turns back our attention. Just like Peter, it's when our eyes meet those of Jesus' that we're broken—in heart and in spirit—and His work through us truly begins.

—Peña

Pastor's Point

1. Have you missed any recent opportunities to share your faith in Christ?
2. If you had it to do over again, what would you do differently?

Today's Prayer

Lord, help me see opportunities to share my faith and make me ready. Don't let me shrink back in fear, but help me boldly stand up for You in even the toughest situations. I know that Your truth always brings life to those who hear.

Walking with Him

Be ready. Make the most of every opportunity to share the love of Jesus and identify with Hm. But if you miss, forget it and get it the next time.

Fitness
Workout #8

Training at a Glance

Because you do reverse crunches last in the workouts, make sure they don't get short shrift as an unwarranted recipient of your "least" effort. It's natural to start dragging as the workout continues, since you're expending a lot of energy through the session. But right before you begin that final exercise, stop for a moment and mentally renew your commitment and give that exercise the same attention you gave the first.

Exercise	Reps Goal	Reps Rd. 1	Reps Rd. 2	Reps Total (2 Rounds)
Plyo push-up				
Standard push-up				
Jump squat				
Crunch				
Reverse crunch				
Rd. time				

Before you begin the exercises, warm up by walking or jogging in place for three to five minutes. Your goal is to perform a total of at least one more rep than you did in your last workout on each exercise and in less total time.

Firm Believer

If you're trying to burn fat and lose weight, try the *PrayFit* plan first thing in the morning. Because your body has essentially been fasting overnight for 8 to 10 hours, training upon awakening allows your body to tap into fat stores for energy. Your body is also burning muscle after the all-night fast, so you should consume about 25 grams of protein to decrease muscle catabolism (breakdown).

Food Byte

Looking for a way to add some color and depth to your dishes? Add healthy fat and creaminess to dips, sandwiches and salads by using avocado, a healthier alternative to mayo.

Walk with the Wise

Faith
The Exercise: Proverbs 13

Have you ever heard the saying "Success breeds success"? Well, the opposite can also be true—failure breeds failure. And the company we choose will have a dramatic effect on which way things go.

The Bible tells us to choose our friends wisely—God knows the influence that friends can have on us, for better and for worse. And as the Proverb says, when we spend a significant amount of time with people, they will influence us.

On the positive side, spending time with people who know more than you or who are better than you at a particular skill makes perfect sense. That's why business leaders have consultants and players have coaches. Let's face it—successful people surround themselves with other highly successful people. They learn from the best and are constantly motivated to excellence.

But the message here is to find people who make wise decisions in life, and spend time with them. Doing this will help you make wise decisions.

Spending time with foolish people—those who make foolish decisions with their money or health or relationships—will not only make you foolish, but you will also suffer harm. In other Bible translations, it says you will be destroyed. That's enough to get my attention.

So find a friend who is walking with God and has successfully created a healthy lifestyle, and start spending time with that person. You will soon be making wise decisions in all areas of your life.

—Page

Pastor's Point

1. Who are you spending substantial time with? Is that person walking with God?
2. Can you trust your friends to be honest with you and build you up?
3. Do they push you to be better and to make wise decisions?
4. Additional reading: 1 John 2:6-11; Deuteronomy 28:9-14.

Today's Prayer

Lord, I pray that You would give me discernment to choose my friends wisely. Help me to connect with people who are walking with You so that I can grow in wisdom.

Walking with Him

Be intentional about spending time with those who have a close relationship with Jesus. And reevaluate some friendships that may be "helping" you make bad choices.

Fitness
Rest

Fitness in Focus: Muscle Fiber Types. There are basically two types of muscle fibers. First, we have slow-twitch muscle fibers. These fibers help with low force production, contract rather slowly, and use fat as their primary source of energy. They also don't fatigue very easily, nor do they grow very easily.

Then, there are fast-twitch muscle fibers. These fibers help produce a lot of force, contract very quickly and rely on glucose rather than depend on fat for energy, as well as creatine phosphate and stored adenosine triphosphate (ATP). And as opposed to their slow-twitch counterparts, they fatigue easily but are good growers when trained with resistance.

Most individuals have close to a 50/50 split of these fiber types throughout their body. Some muscles that are used for posture, such as the abdominals and soleus (deep calf muscle), tend to be slightly higher in slow-twitch muscle fibers, while muscles used for more explosive movements, like the quads, tend to be a bit higher in fast-twitch muscle fibers. Some individuals have a higher percent of slow-twitch muscle fibers in certain muscles, making them able to excel in endurance-type sports such as marathon running and cycling. Other individuals have a higher percentage of fast-twitch muscle fibers in certain muscles, making them able to excel in certain strength and power sports, such as weightlifting and sprinting.

The great thing about the *PrayFit* plan is that it will tax both kinds of muscle fibers because of the balance of intensity each day.

Filled with the Holy Spirit

Faith
The Exercise: John 14:15-26; 16:5-13

Don't you just love how personal Jesus is? Even though He knew that He had to leave His disciples, He assured them that they would never be alone. And He also knew they would need to be filled with power in order to withstand the persecution and suffering they would encounter as they testified to the truth of His resurrection. So many of us receive Christ and are set free from our guilt and shame and sin, but we still try to live life in our own strength. And I have to admit that the thought of giving up control can be a bit scary. As a result, we keep a tight grip on everything—from our relationships to our work and just about everything in between.

God wants so much more for us. He promises us His Holy Spirit. The Spirit is designed to actually live in us and give us truth, wisdom, discernment and power. The great news is that His Spirit never leaves us, but every day we have a choice. We can choose to depend on ourselves or be controlled by His Spirit.

In Acts, the disciples are all filled with His Spirit and power. Their lives were marked with a bold faith and tremendous fruit. When they spoke, people believed in Jesus. When they prayed and worshiped, chains fell off and they were set free from prison. They healed the sick and lame and those tormented by evil spirits.

Something tells me that they walked with confidence. And they definitely weren't worried about what other people thought. Ask God to fill you with His Spirit of truth and power.

—Page

Pastor's Point

1. What do you think of when you hear the word "counselor" (see John 14:15-16)?
2. When seeking God through prayer and the Word, how do we know we can trust what we hear and read (see v. 17)?
3. What role does the Spirit play in our life (see John 14:25-26; 16:13)?
4. Additional reading: 1 Corinthians 6:19-20; Acts 1–4; Ephesians 5:18; Galatians 5.

Today's Prayer

Lord, I pray that I will be filled with Your Spirit—the Holy Spirit of truth and power. Please teach me Your ways as I study Your Word so that I will live each day with confidence and purpose—glorifying You in all that I do.

Walking with Him

Each day we who have believed in Christ are faced with a choice: to take control or to surrender control to God. The tougher choice is to surrender, but it's always the choice that leads to life.

PrayFit Recipe of the Week
Quinoa and Black Bean Salad
with Grilled Shrimp

¾ cup cooked quinoa
¼ cup canned black beans, rinsed and drained
½ cup diced cucumber
¼ cup diced red bell pepper
1 tbsp chopped fresh cilantro
1 tbsp extra virgin olive oil
Lime juice to taste
4 oz. grilled shrimp
Salt and pepper to taste

In a medium-sized bowl, combine quinoa, black beans, cucumber, peppers and cilantro. Drizzle with oil and lime juice, season with salt and pepper and mix well. Serve topped with grilled shrimp.

Calories: 471 | **Protein:** 34 grams | **Carbohydrates:** 45 grams | **Fat:** 18 grams

17

Percent of American children age 2 to 19 who were obese in 2007 and 2008.

Waving Over Walls

Faith
The Exercise: Psalm 145

As a young boy, watching my dad leave for work was more than a habit or tradition—it was a son's ritual. We'd say bye to him at the door, then I'd run to my room and watch for him from my window. I remember that we had a big rock wall over which I could barely see the top of his truck. As he drove down the street he'd wave goodbye out his window and I'd be waving from mine. And all was right with my world.

But boy-oh-boy, if I happened to miss his truck, you'd think the sky had fallen. I still remember the anxiety. "Did I miss him? Did I look down or turn away? As much as I wanted to watch him wave, I needed him to know I was there waving back. And if I thought he didn't see me, I was a mess. Mom would get me on the phone with Dad once he got to work, and he'd calm me down. He'd assure me that he sees me waving, even if I can't see him.

I don't know when I grew out of that, but I didn't outgrow the need to see my dad.

Then I think of my Jesus.

Lord, we're at the window. We've run here to watch You go to work in our world. We're on our tiptoes, and our little eyes are looking for You over the walls of fear and doubt that we ourselves have built. Even if we look down or turn away, You're there. Lord, we need You so much. You see us waving, even if we can't always see You.

—Peña

Pastor's Point

1. Do you call on God when things are going well, or mostly when you need help?
2. Have you felt His nearness in times of loneliness or trouble?

Today's Prayer

Lord, thank You that because of Your presence in my life, I am never alone. You never leave me, and I can talk with You all day long. Help me believe this truth, even when I am lonely or afraid.

Walking with Him

Not only is God near, but also His Spirit lives in us. But He wants us to call on Him all the time, not just when we need help. Today, engage in a conversation with your heavenly Father.

Fitness
Workout #9

Training at a Glance

When you train, it helps to eliminate your distractions. Don't work out in front of a television. Forget whatever happened at work, or that big project you're working on. And don't try to multitask, attempting to get other things done around the house while you're working out. All of those things will ultimately detract from your end-goal results, and you will be less able to fully immerse yourself in the physical experience.

Exercise	Reps Goal	Reps Rd. 1	Reps Rd. 2	Reps Rd. 3	Reps Total (3 Rounds)
Plyo push-up					
Standard push-up					
Decline push-up					
Jump squat					
Bodyweight squat					
Double crunch*					
Reverse crunch*					
Rd. time					

* New exercise

Before you begin the exercises, warm up by walking or jogging in place for three to five minutes. Your goal is to perform a total of at least one more rep than you did in your last workout on each exercise and in less total time.

New Exercise of the Week

Double Crunch
Focus: Upper abs, lower abs

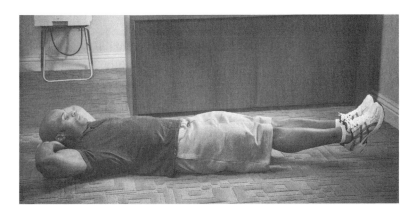

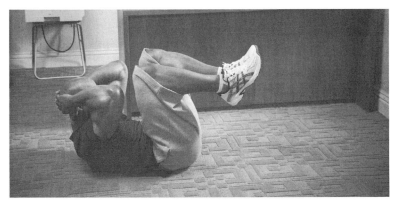

Lie down on the floor with your legs straight, feet together. Place your hands gently behind your head and raise your feet off the floor roughly six inches. Crunch your upper body off the floor while simultaneously bringing your knees toward your torso so that your upper body meets your lower body in the middle. Squeeze and return to the start, allowing your legs to remain above the floor throughout.

Firm Believer

If you're really sore, try taking a short walk—or a jog, if you can stand it—to help circulate blood through stiff, stagnant muscles and loosen them up. Afterwards, take advantage of the elevated blood flow by stretching. You can get a similar effect by sitting in a sauna or hot tub, or simply taking a hot shower.

Food Byte

Put down the sugary sodas and pick up some zero calorie seltzer. If you're a soda drinker, you'll save hundreds of calories per day. Want some flavor? Add lemon, lime, orange, mint or cucumber.

All the Broken Pieces

Faith

The Exercise: 1 Corinthians 14

I've never been very good at riddles. My brain just doesn't work like that. Crosswords? Forget 'em. For the life of me, I can't keep from looking up the answers in the back of the book. But puzzles? Well, that's a different story. My wife, Loretta, and I enjoy a good puzzle.

Shopping for one is easy . . . you just find a cool picture, and that's it. You bring it home, spread the puzzle out on the table, prop up the box cover with the photo on it and get to work. It's not long before what used to be in pieces begins to take the shape of the goal.

But how easy would it be if you took away the box with the picture on it? Tough, right? Or what if you turned off the lights, what then? No wait, I know . . . what if you never saw what the picture was supposed to be in the first place and you turned the lights off? How easy would it be to put that life, I mean, that puzzle together?

For those who are without Christ, that's how life is. They piece together hours, days and weeks, assembling a life without Christ, come what may.

As Christians, our lives are not easily assembled either. Though we have Christ as our picture of perfection, the Bible as our compass and more than enough light for a million-piece life, we still stumble and struggle to put it together. Yet deep inside, we have peace. You know, there are many people around us—at work, at the gym, at school—who try to assemble their life all on their own and they don't have that peace. They're going on feeling alone. In fact, maybe someone you know comes to mind as you read this sentence.

Maybe the only piece of their puzzle that's missing is you. Let's commit to sharing Christ with someone today.

—Peña

Pastor's Point

1. Do you ask God to order your steps and put together all the pieces of your life?
2. Or do you make decisions independent of God?

Today's Prayer

Lord, I can't wait to see the amazing picture that You are creating out of the pieces of my life. Thank You for the peace You give me, because I know that You already see the masterpiece and that You have it all under control. Thank You that I have the Bible as my compass and our conversation as my companion.

Walking with Him

Are you experiencing peace even when the puzzle is still a bunch of jumbled pieces just out of the box? Do you really trust that God has it all under control?

Fitness
Workout #10

Training at a Glance

In the previous "Workout at a Glance" entry, we told you that it's a good idea to eliminate distractions. One thing, however, that's not considered a distraction is music. In fact, listening to music not only serves as a powerful motivator, but it can also help you flush out the outside world. Research has actually shown that those who listen to music during training derive more benefits from their workouts because music enhances focus and helps people "push through the pain" to go longer and get more reps per set. Trying to do more reps each workout—doesn't that sound familiar?

Before you begin the exercises, warm up by walking or jogging in place for three to five minutes. Your goal is to perform a total of at least one more rep than you did in your last workout on each exercise and in less total time.

Exercise	Reps Goal	Reps Rd. 1	Reps Rd. 2	Reps Rd. 3	Reps Total (3 Rounds)
Plyo push-up					
Standard push-up					
Decline push-up					
Jump squat					
Bodyweight squat					
Double crunch					
Reverse crunch					
Rd. time					

Firm Believer

You might not realize how hard your heart is working during exercise. While only about 25 percent oxygen is utilized when a person is resting, this can climb to about 80 percent during exercise. This higher rate equates to more fat burned in the long run.

Food Byte

Instead of going for sugary candy when you have a craving, opt for the natural sweetness of dried fruit. Dried apricots, raisins and figs are also good sources of iron for healthy red blood cells.

United

Faith

The Exercise: Romans 15

One of the things I have always liked about Notre Dame football is the fact that the players don't have their names on the back of their jerseys. There is a sense that when you play for this school, you are part of something far bigger than you. There are decades of history and legendary coaches and miraculous wins.

No one player is more important than the team. It takes commitment, sacrifice and a relentless pursuit of excellence from every single person in the locker room—from the water boys to the head coach, from the athletic trainers to the quarterback.

The same is true for those who are followers of Christ Jesus. No individual believer is more important than the rest of the "team." We are part of a team that has been built on the shoulders of great men and women who sacrificed their very lives for the sake of the gospel—for the truth that Jesus did indeed rise from the dead. The disciples were beheaded, stoned to death and crucified for their faith.

They were willing to pay the ultimate price because they were witnesses of the truth not only of the life of Jesus—with all the miracles and signs—but also of His resurrection.

The Body of Christ is most effective and influential when we are pulling in the same direction and more concerned with God's glory than our own. We are called to connect with each other and be united for a common purpose.

—Page

Pastor's Point

1. Are you more concerned about your own desires or the well-being of your neighbors?
2. In what ways can you unite with other believers to share your faith and influence those around you?
3. Additional reading: Ephesians 4:1-3; Colossians 3:14; Acts 1:1-8.

Today's Prayer

Lord, please give me opportunities to connect with other believers so that we can be united in our quest to share the love of Jesus. Restore damaged relationships so that we can be an example of Your power to bring reconciliation.

Walking with Him

Do you have any unresolved conflict with other believers that is hindering you from working together? Isn't it time to get that resolved? Ask for forgiveness for anything you've done and rejoin the team.

Fitness
Rest

Fitness in Focus: All About Carbs. While protein is the most critical macronutrient for muscle growth, carbohydrates are a close second. Demonized in the media as the cause of fat gain, carbs come in at 4 calories per gram and are a preferred fuel source for hard-working muscles. Naturally, if you consume a high amount of carbohydrate—or protein or fat, for that matter—and don't train to offset that consumption, then increases in fat mass follow. But if you're a *PrayFit* athlete who places a high emphasis on sweat, then you just need a little tweaking to get the most out of this super macronutrient.

Stored in your muscles as glycogen, carbs—with protein—provide fuel for competition and training. If you're training hard, you can go as high as 2 to 3 grams of carbohydrate per pound of bodyweight per day. Of course, if body composition is a concern for you, keep an eye on the mirror and scale back slightly. If your training starts to suffer, however, you should not only return to adequate levels but examine the carb types you're taking in.

For most meals, stick with slow-digesting carbs such as whole grains, sweet potatoes, most fruits and oatmeal. The only times when this is not a hard-and-fast rule are first thing in the morning and post-workout, when your body is carb-deprived. Of course, if you want to take all the guess-work out of the equation, try the *PrayFit* Diet, starting on page 219.

Close Calls

Faith
The Exercise: Luke 17

Growing up in Texas, it was impossible not to be influenced by, or at least exposed to, some good old country music. Because of that, my mind wandered back to my roots yesterday when something I had been expecting, praying and preparing for didn't come to fruition. For reasons out of my control, things just didn't happen. And when I heard the news, I did what any saint would do . . . I flipped out. In that moment, you'd be more likely to find Bigfoot under my bed than to find me exercising faith. Truly, the Tasmanian devil has more self-control.

But after the dust settled from my spinning, a line from an old country song came to mind: "I thank God for unanswered prayers." Because, despite my own agenda, I have no idea what God was protecting me from or what better situation He has in store. As abruptly as I asked, "With God's people praying, how could this happen?" came the answer: It happened because God's people were praying. (Ouch.)

Scoot over, Bigfoot . . .

So, Lord, forgive our unbelief, especially during times of disbelief.

—Peña

Pastor's Point

1. Faith is only faith when it's exercised.
2. Have you experienced disappointment that has made you question God?
3. If so, did it cause you to turn back to Him and trust Him for the future?

Today's Prayer

Lord, help me trust You even when things are tough. Help me believe that You always have my best in mind, especially when I am most disappointed.

Walking with Him

Think of a moment when things didn't go the way you planned. Did it make you anxious and upset or did it drive you back to a simple trust in the loving providence of God?

Fitness
Workout #11

Training at a Glance

Are you finding that sometimes you do more reps in Round 2 or 3 than you got in Round 1? That's just the power of the human spirit. It's why it's considered an advantage to go second in many sporting events, from college football overtime to batting in baseball—once you know what you need to beat, you can prepare yourself mentally for the challenge. Knowing that, is it any wonder why setting specific goals is so powerful, not just in training but in any area of your life? Give a motivated person a finish line, and he or she will find a way to reach it, no matter what.

Exercise	Reps Goal	Reps Rd. 1	Reps Rd. 2	Reps Rd. 3	Reps Total (3 Rounds)
Plyo push-up					
Standard push-up					
Decline push-up					
Jump squat					
Bodyweight squat					
Double crunch					
Reverse crunch					
Rd. time					

Before you begin the exercises, warm up by walking or jogging in place for three to five minutes. Your goal is to perform a total of at least one

more rep than you did in your last workout on each exercise and in less total time.

Firm Believer

Being even slightly dehydrated can impair mental function and focus as well as physical performance. That's because our bodies are about 70 percent water, and water helps with so many bodily functions. The Institute of Medicine (IOM) recommends that men consume 16 cups of water daily and women consume 11 cups of water daily.

Food Byte

Use ground turkey instead of beef for lighter and healthier burgers. Always choose turkey breast meat for the most protein and least saturated fat. Add some onions, garlic and chili powder for a super moist and tasty burger.

Lifetime Achievement

Faith
The Exercise: Matthew 25

Awards season is a fun time around our household. We enjoy watching the Golden Globes, the SAGs, People's Choice and especially the Oscars.

Many of these special shows have their own version of a Lifetime Achievement Award, where a peer is recognized and celebrated for just what the title suggests—a lifelong body of work and the ultimate achievement in show business. What's interesting is that this person is someone who has dedicated his or her life to either pretending to be someone he/she isn't or helping others do the same. Great pretenders.

And when they make their way to the stage, they're greeted with a long embrace from a worthy peer and a standing ovation that seems to last forever. And while there are usually dozens of roles they've played, there's usually one for which they're most remembered.

As believers, we don't earn awards and hear applause for our great performances. Instead, we live our life and offer all our awards to Jesus as a gift for what He has done for us. If someone were to roll tape of our greatest hits and most celebrated performances, they'd all have one main character: Jesus. There's nothing good in us but Him. And if we act as if there is, we're not only pretending for others but we're fooling ourselves. And make no mistake, when our life is through and He welcomes us home with an embrace, there will be applause . . . from us.

—Peña

Pastor's Point

1. Are you living in a way that brings glory to Jesus, or for personal awards and applause?

2. What things might need to change for you to be called a good and faithful servant?

Today's Prayer

Lord, forgive me for seeking the applause and awards of men. I offer my life to You as a living sacrifice. Make everything I do a right reflection of You.

Walking with Him

What are some things you can do behind the scenes to serve others that no one but God will ever know about? Anonymous giving, serving, fasting and praying can go a long way to make your heart right.

Fitness
Workout #12

Training at a Glance

You're certainly developing expertise on all of these exercises, but it can't hurt to revisit a couple of key pointers to ensure your form isn't faltering. On your push-ups, is your butt sagging? On your squats, are you landing hard with your knees locked out? And on your crunches, are you tugging at your head with your hands as you rep? If the answer is yes on any of the above, take this opportunity to make the appropriate corrections.

Exercise	Reps Goal	Reps Rd. 1	Reps Rd. 2	Reps Rd. 3	Reps Total (3 Rounds)
Plyo push-up					
Standard push-up					
Decline push-up					
Jump squat					
Bodyweight squat					
Double crunch					
Reverse crunch					
Rd. time					

Before you begin the exercises, warm up by walking or jogging in place for three to five minutes. Your goal is to perform a total of at least one

more rep than you did in your last workout on each exercise and in less total time.

Firm Believer

Besides being important for your health, research finds that drinking water can enhance fat loss. German researchers reported that drinking about 2 cups of cold water on an empty stomach boosted metabolic rate by 30 percent. The scientists estimated that if you drink 2 cups of cold water before breakfast, lunch and dinner every day for a year, you'd burn almost 17,500 extra calories, which translates into a little more than 5 pounds of body fat.

Food Byte

Keep your cholesterol low with oatmeal. Oats are high in soluble fiber, which keeps you full longer and helps remove cholesterol from the body. Oatmeal is a great way to start your day with lasting fuel.

Worthless

Faith
The Exercise: Acts 20

When is the last time you thought, *My life is worth nothing*? I mean this in the sense that you count your life here as nothing unless you have Jesus. In a culture that emphasizes boosting one's self-esteem, and where everyone wins because we don't want to hurt anybody's feelings, this is not a popular theme.

And then we see athletes pointing to their name on the jersey or thumping their chests when they make a great play. Still others refuse to play for their team because they don't have a chance of winning a championship. It is the ultimate in selfishness.

We have plenty of examples of the "It's all about me" belief in sports and in life. After all, there's no *I* in "team," but there is an *M* and an *E*.

But Paul continues to throw selfish pursuits under the bus. In the face of trials and suffering, he doesn't demand to be traded so he can win a ring. He doesn't plead with God for an easy way out or for a simple assignment or for prosperity. You get the sense that comfort and convenience are not even distant thoughts to Paul.

Paul, like you and me, was on a mission. He realized that finishing the race meant being faithful to his Lord Jesus and the truth of His resurrection. He gave up his "right" to a life of status and wealth and personal gain; apart from Jesus, his life was worth nothing to him.

Paul also knew that his personal résumé of great knowledge and education, family connections and status were empty and useless without Jesus. We often hold on to the things of this life so tightly because we wrongly think this is all there is. The things of this world are passing away.

It's time to give ourselves fully to things that will last forever.

—Page

Pastor's Point

1. Do you major on looking out for your own interests?
2. Or like Paul, can you say that your life apart from finishing your mission with Jesus is worth nothing?
3. Additional reading: Galatians 2:20; Philippians 3:7-11; Philippians 1:21.

Today's Prayer

Lord, I pray that You would take away my selfishness and that I would focus instead on the needs of others. Help me to intentionally put the needs of others ahead of my own.

Walking with Him

Do something unselfish for someone else today. Maybe even share your faith. Be intentional and anticipate the needs of others. Go above and beyond as you serve.

Fitness
Rest

Fitness in Focus: Know Your Fats. Fats are the third and final macronutrient, and just like carbs and protein, they play their own special role in the body. Some of fats' important jobs include hormone production, nervous system function, shock absorption in joints and temperature regulation. Like carbohydrates, fats are also burned for energy during different intensity levels of exercise.

Fat has gotten a bad reputation for causing weight gain, but the truth is, eating the right kinds of fat in the right amounts can actually help you lose weight more easily. As with protein, it takes your body longer to digest fat than carbohydrates. This keeps you feeling satisfied and gives you longer-lasting energy after a meal. But keep in mind that fats are a more concentrated source of calories—a gram of fat has more calories than a gram of carbs or protein (9 as opposed to 4 with carbs and protein), which means that portions need to stay in check to make sure your overall calories don't get out of control.

It's important to recognize that there are small amounts of saturated fats in healthy foods like milk, cheese, meats and fish, but this doesn't make them "bad" foods, as they also contain healthy components like protein, calcium, vitamins and heart-healthy fats. It does mean, however, that you need to pick and choose where these foods should fit into your diet. You should seek all these good nutrients, but you should also moderate your intake of saturated fats and calories to keep your weight under control and your heart healthy. Trans fats, on the other hand, offer little or no healthful benefits and should be avoided as much as possible.

Saturated Fats

fatty meats	cheese	cocoa butter
butter	lard	coconut oil
whole milk	ice cream	palm kernel oil

Trans Fats

Commercially prepared baked goods like cookies, cakes and pies
Snack foods like chips and crackers
Some fried foods like donuts and certain brands of French fries
Some brands of peanut butter
Anything with "partially hydrogenated oils" on the label

10.4

Percent increase in obesity among children ages 2 to 5 between 1976–1980 and 2007–2008.

Connected to the Vine

Faith
The Exercise: John 15:1-17

A few weeks back, I woke up and started my morning routine. I turned on the water to brush my teeth and immediately noticed the absence of—you guessed it—water! Since we're on a well, I figured I'd be able to diagnose the problem pretty quickly. So after the professionals came and gave me the $2,500 estimate to replace the well pump, I decided to fix it myself.

Three days later, I realized why plumbers get paid so much for what they do. I had enlisted the help of my brother and several neighbors, and we had spent two evenings working long after dark. After we got the new well pump connected, we tested it before we lowered it the 240 feet to the bottom of the well. This turned out to be a smart idea, especially since the new pump didn't work. We finally discovered that the problem was in the electrical connection.

When we get disconnected from the Vine––when we lose our daily connection to Jesus—we don't work either. In fact, Jesus tells us that we can't accomplish anything apart from Him. But when we are connected to Him, and we accept His pruning, we will produce much fruit. Isn't that really what you want—a life that makes a difference for eternity? Then, staying connected to Jesus to start each day is the most important thing you can do.

—Page

Pastor's Point

1. What do you need to do to connect with God to grow spiritually?
2. What does Jesus mean when He says that apart from Him you can do nothing (see John 15:5)?
3. When Jesus talks about bearing fruit, what does that look like in your life (see v. 5)?
4. Additional reading: Psalms 1:1-3; 92:12-15; Galatians 5:22.

Today's Prayer

Lord, I pray that I will always remain connected to You through prayer and time spent in Your Word. Help me to understand the benefits of being pruned so that I can bear much fruit.

Walking with Him

There is nothing more important than your connection with God. It is the only way that you can be filled, empowered and controlled by the Holy Spirit. Otherwise, everything you do is in your own strength, and you are destined to be worn out by the stress of life. Make the connection today.

PrayFit Recipe of the Week
Spicy Turkey Burgers

5 oz. ground turkey breast
1 tbsp minced red onion
1 tbsp chopped roasted red pepper
1/8 tsp chili powder
pinch salt
1 slice low-fat Swiss cheese
2 cups mixed greens
2 tsp olive oil
Freshly squeezed lemon juice to taste

Preheat grill or grill pan. In a medium bowl combine turkey, onion, roasted pepper, chili power and salt; mix and form into a burger. Cook for 4 to 5 minutes per side until cooked through. Top with Swiss cheese and serve over mixed greens dressed with olive oil and lemon juice.

Calories: 324 calories | **Protein:** 44 grams | **Carbohydrates:** 7 grams | **Fat:** 11 grams

80

Percent of children who were overweight at 10 to 15 years of age and who ended up obese at age 25.

A Profession of Faith

Faith
The Exercise: Mark 12:44

Typically, in New Testament times, when people gave to the treasury, they announced it loudly for all to hear, grabbing the attention of anyone within earshot. But who would notice a frail widow giving only two coins? Nobody . . . right? But when two coins are all you have, when it's your life you're offering, the sound it makes gets God's attention.

We don't often have company, but last night our little condo was packed. First, there was the couple who have been married more than 45 years—a sweet-as-can-be combo who act like they're still on their honeymoon. Then, there's the teacher. With her writing and peaceful delivery, she's touched hearts for years. Across from me at the dinner table were the mom and dad who raised two boys and a girl to be godly people and of whom they're so proud; tears filled the dad's eyes as he spoke of them. And on the couch was the missionary. Today, this spirit-filled warrior of a man spends months at a time teaching people in the underground church of the most dangerous, inaccessible areas of Asia. And finally, there was my preacher. For more than 40 years he led churches, mine included, for the cause of Christ. Because of his ministry, *his confrontational evangelism*, I came to know Jesus as my personal Lord and savior.

The couple, the teacher, the parents, the preacher and the missionary—many experiences, but only two human beings. You see, all of these life experiences refer to Henry and Sandie Powell—two people who have lived their whole life to give their whole life.

Do I live that way? Is my life an offering? Is yours? God might not be calling us to be missionaries, but He's calling us somewhere.

—Peña

Pastor's Point

1. Like the widow in Mark 12:43-44, are you willing to give everything you've got as you follow the Lord?
2. What might need to change in order for that to happen?
3. Additional reading: 2 Corinthians 9:6-12.

Today's Prayer

Here I am, Lord. Here are my two coins of work, of school, of family and health. They're Yours. All I have I give to You today. Take my life as an offering.

Walking with Him

Let go. We all have a deeply human compulsion to hold on to those two coins. It is survival instinct mixed in with a bit of selfishness and doubt. But today, it's time to let go—whether it's a grudge you've held with someone or a heavy yoke of guilt that's been weighing you down. You may find that once you liberate yourself and trust the Lord, He can use you for great things.

Fitness
Workout #13: Baseline, Week 3

Training at a Glance

The new recruit this week? The plank. Unlike every other exercise you've done in this program, the plank is a static (otherwise known as isometric) move, in that you hold a position for as long as you can. Instead of building your strength dynamically through movement, it increases your strength by calling upon your muscles to stay rigid, which as you'll find can be just as tough.

Before you begin the exercises, warm up by walking or jogging in place for three to five minutes.

Exercise	Reps Goal	Reps Rd. 1	Reps Rd. 2	Reps Rd. 3	Reps Rd. 4	Reps Total (4 Rounds)
Plyo push-up						
Standard push-up						
Decline push-up						
Jump squat						
Bodyweight squat						
Lunge						
Double crunch						
Reverse crunch						
Crunch						
Rd. time						
Plank time*						

* New exercise. The plank time is not a part of the timed workout, but rather your goal is to hold the plank for as long as possible, noting the time. Your total time will then be your goal to beat the next day.

New Exercise of the Week

Plank
Focus: Core

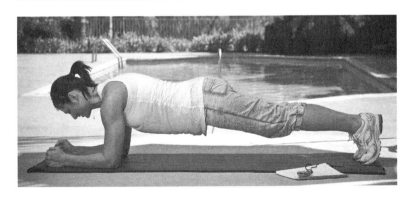

Get on all fours on the floor with your elbows directly under your shoulders. Extend your legs and flex your ankles so that your toes touch the floor and your heels push straight back. Keep your abs pulled in tight, leg muscles contracted and back flat. Support your bodyweight on your forearms, elbows and toes. Your body should create a straight line from your shoulders to your heels.

Firm Believer

Hitting your *PrayFit* exercises before breakfast may help you burn more fat. Overnight, your body uses stored sugar (carbs) as fuel for your organs. When you awake from what is essentially an overnight fast, your body tends to use fat as its preferred fuel source.

Food Byte

Complex carbohydrates take longer to digest and provide a more steady delivery of energy. These kinds of carbs typically contain good amounts of hunger-fighting fiber and various vitamins and minerals. Complex carbs are found in legumes (beans, peas and lentils), starchy vegetables and whole grain cereals and breads. Fruits and vegetables contain a combination of simple and complex carbs, and they also pack in a ton of vitamins and minerals relative to their low number of calories, which makes them perfect for getting in all of your vital nutrients while trying to lose weight.

On the Rock

Faith
The Workout: Psalm 62

Early morning waves captivated me, and I found myself walking along the shore, gathering my thoughts and goals for the day. After about a mile or so, I came upon this huge, coral-like rock that was sitting halfway in the water and halfway on the sand. It was awesome. So, of course, I started climbing.

Once on top, I felt a sense of accomplishment, despite the fact that I'd only climbed a whopping six feet. With hands on hips, I stood there in hero's stance. And when my moment of triumph was over, I started down, but then realized that I'd been standing on literally thousands of little crablike creatures, probably half an inch long. Their shells were hard as granite. And as I reached down to grab one of them, it moved slightly with a sort of twisting motion. And when it moved, so did I . . . fast.

Gathering my wits, I knelt down for closer inspection, and each time I reached for them, they'd twist. I soon realized that what they were doing was clinging to the rock as my foreign hand approached. They held so tightly that it took effort on my part to pull them away. It didn't take me long to figure out that they held on to the rock as a protective mechanism against the crashing waves so they wouldn't easily drift away. Smart crabs. They knew the meaning of stronghold. As the waves heightened, they tightened.

If only I did the same.

—Peña

Pastor's Point

1. When life gets tough, what do you cling to? Do you just work harder or do you hold on to the hand of God?
2. When the waves crash against you, will you stand because you have your foundation on God's Word?

Today's Prayer

Lord, when the storms of life come and the waves crash down on me, help me hang on to You and the truth of Your Word. You are my Rock and my Salvation.

Walking with Him

The one who builds his house on the rock—on God's principles and faith in Jesus—will withstand the storms of life. The one who builds on sand— on his or her own strength and gifts and ideas—will fall with a crash. The tougher things get, the tighter we need to hold on.

Fitness
Workout #14

Training at a Glance

The groupings in this week's workouts—the three types of push-ups, the three leg exercises, and the three abdominal crunch variations—are valuable to remember after you've finished your *PrayFit* program. That's because, as you move on to other workouts or activities, you can return to them again and again as a way to warm up your body for action. They are synergistic, powerful exercise trios that can always be easily added to any workout program you may undertake in the future.

Before you begin the exercises, warm up by walking or jogging in place for three to five minutes. With the exception of the plank, your goal is to perform a total of at least one more rep than you did in your last workout on each exercise and in less total time.

Exercise	Reps Goal	Reps Rd. 1	Reps Rd. 2	Reps Rd. 3	Reps Rd. 4	Reps Total (4 Rounds)
Plyo push-up						
Standard push-up						
Decline push-up						
Jump squat						
Bodyweight squat						
Lunge						
Double crunch						
Reverse crunch						
Crunch						
Rd. time						
Plank time*						

* The plank time is not a part of the timed workout, but rather your goal is to hold the plank for as long as possible, noting the time. Your total time will then be your goal to beat the next day.

Firm Believer

Looking to add to your day's exercise bounty? Try isometric holds. Isometrics pit your muscles against immovable objects—like a wall, a pole or each other. Next time you're at a stoplight or in front of the TV, try pressing your hands together in front of your chest for 30 seconds, breathing normally along the way. Rest for 30 to 60 seconds and repeat 3 to 4 more times. This prompts an intense contraction in your chest and shoulder muscles, adding to the work you put in during today's workout. Isometrics can be done anywhere but should only be used to supplement a workout routine replete with normal isotonic movements like the ones prescribed here. Go to prayfit.com for more information on isometric holds.

Food Byte

Fats are a more concentrated source of calories—a gram of fat has more calories than a gram of carbs or protein, which means that portions need to stay in check to make sure your overall calories don't get out of control.

Drop the Weight

Faith
The Exercise: Hebrews 12

Every competitive athlete is looking for an edge—a way to get bigger, faster or stronger.

In the training room, we often have athletes wear a weighted vest as they go through their drills. It helps the athletes to push beyond their normal limits. It adds stress to their body in a controlled environment to prepare them for the intense demands of competition. And when the vest comes off, these athletes often feel invincible. They are faster and stronger and more agile than they could have imagined. It's as if we have set a prisoner free!

But if I were to tell you that you had to wear that 40-pound vest in the game, you would think I was crazy. There's no way that you would be able to perform at your best. You would be slower and become fatigued very early in the contest. And you would be much more susceptible to injury as the game wore on. The additional weight would destroy your performance.

In Hebrews 12:1, we are encouraged to "lay aside every weight, and the sin which so easily ensnares us" (*NKJV*). Sin is heavy. It weighs us down and trips us up. It is the spiritual equivalent of wearing a weighted vest into competition. The author of Hebrews realized that sin causes us to lose strength. It wears us out so that we are unable to finish the race with endurance. It tangles us up. It makes us far less effective in carrying out our mission.

But when we confess our sins to Almighty God, we are set free. We feel clean and courageous and confident. We feel invincible. A heavy heart weighed down by sin brings us down. But a clean heart that has been forgiven lifts us up. It is time to drop the weight.

—Page

Pastor's Point

1. Is there sin in your life that is weighing you down?
2. Can you see the ways that sin is hurting you as you walk with Christ?
3. Are you willing to confess those sins and be set free?
4. Additional reading: 1 Corinthians 9:24; Hebrews 10:35-36.

Today's Prayer

Lord, I pray that You would expose the sin in my life that is weighing me down and that I would repent and get right with You.

Walking with Him

If you are feeling heavy, you are probably trying to carry the burdens of life on your own shoulders. God asks us to cast our cares on Him because He cares for us (see 1 Pet. 5:7). Confess your sin and restore your relationship with Him.

Fitness
Rest

Fitness in Focus: Packed with Protein. As you already know from being on the *PrayFit* diet plan, protein is a critical component to your health and success. The main function of protein in the body is to build and maintain muscle to keep you lean and strong. Protein is also involved in numerous chemical reactions to regulate metabolism and keep cells healthy. Unlike carbs, which are all about energy production, protein is more about structure. Carbohydrates provide the energy needed to make sure muscle cells scoop up protein and (along with exercise) convert it into lean body mass (aka muscles). Protein is also digested differently than carbs; the structural pieces of protein take longer to digest, so they tend to keep you full for longer.

Lean vs. Fatty Sources of Protein: When it comes to protein, the leaner the source, the better. Sure, heavily marbled cuts of meat have protein, but they also come loaded with high amounts of artery-clogging saturated fat, cholesterol and extra calories. Stick to lean meats like chicken and turkey breast, pork tenderloin and lean cuts of beef. Fish is also lower in fat and calories yet packed with healthy protein. Dairy is a good protein source too, so make room in your diet for eggs, nonfat milk and yogurt. There are also some great vegetarian sources of protein, like beans, legumes and whole grains

34

Percent of American adults age 20 and over who were obese in 2005–2006.

Wilson!

Faith
The Exercise: Luke 18

In the movie *Cast Away,* Tom Hanks's character, Chuck Noland, was a time-obsessed FedEx analyst with a simple job: deliver the mail on time. After his plane crashed, he got washed up on a deserted island where he spent four lonely years. Well, he wasn't totally alone.

Wilson, a volleyball that Chuck found in the wreckage, became more like a friend than a piece of sporting goods equipment. Clearly out of his mind, Chuck would talk and even argue with the ball. But when he finally escaped from the island, his raft was hit by a storm. And when he woke up, he realized Wilson had been thrown overboard (cue the sad music). After attempts to retrieve Wilson failed, a heartbroken Chuck realized he couldn't take it with him. He knew he had to decide: be saved or go in after his prized possession.

Silly, right? I mean, who in his right mind would act that way? When I saw that scene, I was shaking my head, thinking, *It's a volleyball, you nut!* But then I thought of the rich young ruler and the answer Jesus gave him. Haven't we all been in that boat? Ever gone overboard on stuff? Funny, like watching Chuck, I wonder if the Lord ever shakes His head at how crazy we get about our toys.

—Peña

Pastor's Point

1. In what ways have you let stuff get in the way of your relationship with God?
2. What are you holding on to that you are unwilling to let go of?

Today's Prayer

Lord, remove anything in me that keeps me from You. The choice is an easy one, and I choose You.

Walking with Him

We often don't understand the value of what Jesus actually did for us. Because if we did, we'd give up everything to get what He gives. Eternal life is worth more than all the money in the world or all the toys we can accumulate. Yet we hold on so tightly to our material possessions. Don't let anything come between you and Jesus.

Fitness
Workout #15

Training at a Glance

Because the double crunch is basically a crunch and reverse crunch combined, you'll certainly be taxed as you complete the double and move on to the reverse and the regular versions. Embrace the intense burn you feel as you do the reverse crunch and crunch, and let it build to a point where you feel you cannot complete another rep. Then do one more, as that will be your most productive rep of the day.

Exercise	Reps Goal	Reps Rd. 1	Reps Rd. 2	Reps Rd. 3	Reps Rd. 4	Reps Total (4 Rounds)
Plyo push-up						
Standard push-up						
Decline push-up						
Jump squat						
Bodyweight squat						
Lunge						
Double crunch						
Reverse crunch						
Crunch						
Rd. time						
Plank time*						

* The plank time is not a part of the timed workout, but rather your goal is to hold the plank for as long as possible, noting the time. Your total time will then be your goal to beat the next day.

Before you begin the exercises, warm up by walking or jogging in place for three to five minutes. With the exception of the plank, your goal is to perform a total of at least one more rep than you did in your last workout on each exercise and in less total time.

Firm Believer

Protein contains 4 calories per gram. So a medium-sized chicken breast containing 40 grams of protein (roughly 6 ounces) gives you 160 calories from protein alone. (Note: 2 grams of fat runs the calorie total of the breast to roughly 178.)

Food Byte

A complete protein is composed of 20 different amino acids. Some are more critical than others. At the top of the list are the BCAAs (branched chain amino acids), which include leucine, isoleucine and valine. Arginine is crucial for helping production of nitric oxide (NO), which dilates blood vessels, taking more nutrients to muscles during workouts. Glutamine is also high on the list because it keeps muscle protein synthesis high and breakdown low and helps to boost your immune system.

Total Recall

Faith
The Workout: Matthew 27

Sender would like to recall the previous message . . .

You've probably seen that note in your inbox from time to time. And while it always strikes me as funny to receive it (seeing as I've already read the message), I can definitely relate to the person who sent it. How many times have I said something that I wanted to quickly retract? Even if I felt I had the right to sound off, I often want to hit the recall button and take it all back. Unfortunately, the damage I caused with my big mouth is already done.

> Now Jesus stood before the governor. And the governor asked Him, saying, "Are You the King of the Jews?" Jesus said to him, "It is as you say." And while He was being accused by the chief priests and elders, He answered nothing. Then Pilate said to Him, "Do You not hear how many things they testify against You?" But He answered him not one word, so that the governor marveled greatly (Matt. 27:11-14, *NKJV*).

If anyone had the right to speak up in his own defense, Jesus did. When He was being unfairly charged as a criminal, He could have breathed a small hurricane or whispered a call for the angels to flank His side, but He didn't. He was innocent of all charges, yet our hopeless calls for help left Him speechless, and our fate was sealed with His lips.

So today, let's challenge ourselves to hold our tongue, even when nobody would blame us. And when the urge to show teeth in anger overwhelms, let's remember that lions don't have to roar.

Jesus the lamb taught us that.

—Peña

Pastor's Point

1. Have you ever said anything you wish you could take back?
2. How hard was it to make it right with the person you hurt?
3. Do you find it difficult to hold your tongue and not respond when under attack?

Today's Prayer

Lord, You know that the tongue has the power of life and death. And my words can determine the direction of my life. Help me to be careful with the words I speak so that I bring life to those who hear.

Walking with Him

Don't defend yourself. Let God do it. Resist the temptation to strike back when you've been offended or hurt. In fact, do the opposite—give a kind word in the face of anger or opposition. Bless those who curse you, and you will be blessed.

Fitness
Workout #16

Training at a Glance

This is it, so give it everything you have, and conclude this program with an effort and a result you can be proud of. (And just by making it this far, and fulfilling the commitment you made to yourself when you began, you definitely have a lot to be proud of.) Every drop of sweat, every ounce of toil, has been for the greater good of forging a bond between your body, mind and soul.

Before you begin the exercises, warm up by walking or jogging in place for three to five minutes. With the exception of the plank, your goal is to perform a total of at least one more rep than you did in your last workout on each exercise and in less total time.

Exercise	Reps Goal	Reps Rd. 1	Reps Rd. 2	Reps Rd. 3	Reps Rd. 4	Reps Total (4 Rounds)
Plyo push-up						
Standard push-up						
Decline push-up						
Jump squat						
Bodyweight squat						
Lunge						
Double crunch						
Reverse crunch						
Crunch						
Rd. time						
Plank time*						

* The plank time is not a part of the timed workout, but rather your goal is to hold the plank for as long as possible, noting the time. Your total time will then be your goal to beat the next day.

Firm Believer

As you conclude your *PrayFit* workouts today, it's important to think ahead to where you'll take your newfound strength and fitness next. Having gone through these two months of progressive workouts, your body may need a break. That's fine. Take one week off from exercise, then get back after it.

At PrayFit.com, we provide daily fitness tips to help you find your next level as well as nutritional tips to support your progress. Maybe you'll choose to enter a race of some kind or try your hand at pushing more weight at your local gym, or you can always go back and repeat this entire program. Whatever your choice, we hope you've become stronger, inside and out, with *PrayFit*.

He's Got Your Back

Faith
The Exercise: Ephesians 6

It has been said that life is not a playground; it's a battleground. And if you spend any time reading the Old Testament, you will realize that our God is a righteous "warrior." Most of the battles happen in the unseen world of angels and demons and then play out in the physical world that we see.

Knowing this, God gives us very clear instruction on how to be prepared for the battle. He lists six important weapons that make up our spiritual armor. All six—the belt of truth, the breastplate of righteousness, the shoes of peace, the shield of faith, the helmet of salvation, and the sword of the Spirit—protect you from frontline attack. Not one piece of armor provides protection for your back.

In fact, we are instructed in Philippians 3:13 to "[Forget] what is behind and [strain] toward what is ahead." We are told to press on. Never look back. There's no reason to look back. God has your back. He gives us no armor for our backside because He has it covered. When we live according to the Spirit, when we are right with God, when we confess our sins and are clean, we have nothing to fear. In Proverbs 3:24, Solomon tells us that when we use good judgment, our sleep will be sweet. In other words, we don't have to worry about anything coming back to haunt us or catch up with us.

Ask Peyton Manning of the Indianapolis Colts how important his left tackle is. He literally can drop back in the pocket and never worry about getting hit from behind. He can keep his vision down field to attack the defense. When you have that assurance, that confidence, you can perform at the highest levels! Rest assured—God has your back!

—Page

Pastor's Point

1. Are you surprised that God did not give you specific armor to protect your back?
2. Can you fully trust that God will protect you from unseen danger and calamity?
3. Have you been able to forget the past, even when things didn't go your way, and continue advancing against the enemy?
4. Additional reading: Proverbs 3:21-26; Philippians 3; Ephesians 6.

Today's Prayer

Lord, I put on Your spiritual armor today so that I can take my stand against the schemes of the devil. Thank You for protecting my back as I advance and walk with You.

Walking with Him

Get ready for war. We need to get serious about the war that rages in the spiritual world. The only way to fight is to put on His armor. Read the Word. Pray. Get ready.

Fitness
Rest

Fitness in Focus: Learning Labels. Cruising through a supermarket can be daunting when you're trying to revamp your nutritional habits. You know you need to eat healthier, and you have a general idea of the types of foods you should be eating, but invariably, and instinctively, you end up looking at labels. Your brain (and your gut) wants to do its own investigating, and that's fine—if you know what you're looking for. Try these eight tips the next time you're hit with the urge to peek at a label.

1. **Serving Size:** Check the serving size so you know what a proper portion should be. Some foods are deceptively packaged to include more (or less) of what you think you're getting. A bottle of Gatorade, for example, isn't a single serving—it's at least two

servings, if not more—so you have to double the ingredients on the label to get your actual net intake.

2. **Say No to Trans Fat:** When it comes to fat, choose foods that are low in saturated fat and free of trans fats; look for healthy mono- and polyunsaturated fats.

3. **Fat Finder:** Even if a food has less than 0.5 gram of fat per serving, the label can read 0 grams—check the ingredient list for the "hidden" fats, particularly if you're watching your caloric intake. Fat is the most calorically dense macronutrient, weighing in at 9 calories per fat gram.

4. **Go High Fiber**: Choose high-fiber grains, breads and cereals for your diet. These slower-digesting, heart-healthy carbs are a great source of energy and don't have the same detrimental effect on blood sugar as other processed carbs. Look for foods with 3 grams or more of fiber per serving. As a bonus, for every gram of fiber, you can subtract that from the carb total for your lower "net carbs" number.

5. **What is HFCS?** You will want to choose foods without processed sweeteners like high fructose corn syrup. HFCS has little to no nutritional value and can, over time, have adverse effects on blood sugar and body composition—not to mention your teeth.

6. **Wholly Goodness:** Make sure grains are "whole" (whole wheat, whole-grain oats, and so forth). This ensures you're getting the least processed version of this must-have food.

7. **Hidden Sugar:** Added sugars go by many names and are, without question, worth avoiding. Look for the names corn syrup, molasses, evaporated cane juice, brown sugar and invert sugar (and check out a complete list of "hidden sugar" names on the Web). Keep those out of your grocery cart!

8. Convenience Hurts: Avoid high-sodium processed foods like frozen dinners and packaged snacks. These easy-to-prepare and easy-to-eat foods come at a price and should be avoided altogether if you have problems with elevated blood pressure.

12.9
Percent of private insurance spending related to obesity.

Pleasing to God

Faith
The Exercise: Genesis 39:1-6

Joseph was well acquainted with adversity. He also knew what it was like to go through things that were beyond his control. His father, Jacob, loved him more than all of his brothers and did not conceal his favoritism. As a result, his brothers resented Joseph to the point that they were willing to kill him. Instead, they sold him into slavery. Joseph went from "golden boy" to slave almost overnight. And Joseph was at a crossroads. Would he be angry and bitter at God for the situation he was in, or would he humbly submit and surrender to God's sovereign plan? Adversity has a strange way of bringing clarity.

Joseph chose to surrender. He chose obedience and discovered that if he were to survive, he would need to accept both the good and bad and rely on the power and presence of God. His words and actions and attitudes all pointed to the power of his God. The Lord prospered him and gave him success in everything he did; the presence of God was so prevalent in his life that everyone was able to see it.

You see, God loves when we choose to follow Him—when our hearts are His and we obey His voice. "For the eyes of the Lord range throughout the earth to strengthen those whose hearts are fully committed to him" (2 Chron. 16:9). This is what makes a life that is pleasing to God. Will you be like Joseph?

—Page

Pastor's Point

1. What trials are you facing? How can you respond in a God-pleasing way, like Joseph?
2. In what ways can you surrender the outcome to God?

Today's Prayer

Lord, I pray that You will prepare me for the adversities I will face. Solidify my commitment to You no matter how difficult life becomes so that I will be a light that everyone will see, to Your glory.

Walking with Him

Life can be tough, and adversity is almost guaranteed. Even though we can't prepare for every challenge we'll face, we can trust our Guide, no matter what. And trusting God means that as we continue to do the right thing, we can enjoy peace, because it's all in His hands. Do the right thing even when things aren't going the way you planned.

PrayFit Recipe of the Week
Guacamole Dip

½ avocado, diced
¼ cup steamed (shelled) edamame
¼ cup chopped tomato
1 tsp lime juice
Salt and pepper to taste
10 baby carrot sticks

Combine first five ingredients in a medium bowl and mash well with a fork. For a smoother dip, combine ingredients in a food processor fitted with a steel blade and pulse until dip reaches desired consistency. Serve with baby carrot sticks.

Calories: 234 calories | **Protein:** 7 grams | **Carbohydrates:** 21 grams | **Fat:** 15 grams

34
Percent of men 18 and older who were engaged in regular leisure-time physical activity in 2008.

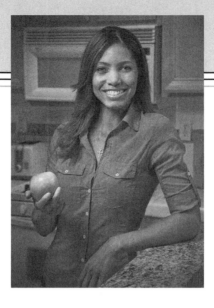

PrayFit: Eating in Balance

By Jim Stoppani, PhD

*Then God said, "I give you every seed-bearing plant on the face of
the whole earth and every tree that has fruit with seed in it. They will be yours
for food. And to all the beasts of the earth and all the birds of the air
and all the creatures that move on the ground—everything that has
the breath of life in it—I give every green plant for food." And it was so.*

GENESIS 1:29-30

The Lord blessed us with myriad foods from which to choose for physical nourishment. Unfortunately, He also inspired us with the ability to concoct dishes that are calorically dense and physically damaging—even if they're better tasting. Not surprisingly, that gift came after Eve ate from the tree in the Garden of Eden!

Somewhere along the line, food, while essential to our vitality, became our worst enemy. Here in America, eateries have been slowly polluting our collective health by way of king-sized portions and menus that are riddled with potentially health-threatening ingredients.

The result is a nation with its health on the decline. A million "quick fix" diets—many of which you probably saw to the left and right of this book when you bought it—have deluded us into thinking that a better body is one crash week away. The truth is much more humbling, but ultimately easier to sustain. Friends, it is in balance that you will find the miracle of long-term healthy living and a physique that is stronger for the journey.

Deeper Study:
Macronutrients

The *PrayFit* diet platform is based on an equal percent of total calories from protein, carbohydrates and fat—33 percent of each across the board. This not only makes the diet easy to remember, but it ensures that you are taking in a well-balanced diet that provides adequate amounts of quality protein for repair and regeneration of tissues, healthy sources of carbohydrates for energy, and healthy fats for proper brain function, cardiovascular health and joint function.

> **Calorie:**
> The energy needed to increase the temperature of 1 gram of water by 1° C.

When these three macronutrients are eaten in equal quantities (and in proper amounts), fat loss is optimized while important muscle tissue is spared. In addition, research shows that when protein and carbs are eaten in equal amounts, brain function is optimized, allowing you to be more efficient at work and on all cognitive tasks, such as your daily devotionals. This is due to the fact that such a diet better maintains steady blood glucose and insulin levels throughout the day. The maintenance of steady blood glucose and insulin levels with the PrayFit nutrition plan will also help to prevent disorders such as type 2 diabetes and cardiovascular disease.

On the *PrayFit* diet you will eat approximately 33 percent of your total calories from protein, 33 percent from carbohydrates and 33 percent from fat each day. Or for grams, that equates to 1 gram of protein per pound of bodyweight, 1 gram of carbohydrate per pound of bodyweight and about 0.5 grams of fat per pound of bodyweight. For a 150-pound person, that equals 150 grams of protein, 150 grams of carbohydrates, and 75 grams of fat. This comes to about 12 calories per pound of bodyweight, or about 1,800 calories for the 150-pound person.

PrayFit Protein

Protein is a critical element of the *PrayFit* diet (or any diet for that matter). Dietary protein is necessary for the repair and regeneration of almost all tissues in the body, which is even more vital when starting a new exercise program or adding new challenges to an existing routine. It's also critical for making the functional proteins that perform important jobs in the body. For example, hemoglobin, which carries oxygen in the blood to the tissues of the body, is a protein, as is the hormone insulin.

All major meals on the *PrayFit* diet focus on protein as the major staple. For example, at breakfast you could have three egg whites and one whole egg scrambled with a slice of low-fat cheese, along with oatmeal and orange juice, for more than 30 grams of protein.

> **Insulin:**
> An anabolic hormone produced by the pancreas. Insulin provides both positive and negative consequences in the body. The positive is that it allows the body to use glucose for fuel and enhances muscle recovery. The negative is that it can also cause the body to store fat.

Starting your day with a high protein meal is not only important for fueling your muscles, but also your brain. Research from the Swiss Federal Institute of Technology (Zurich) discovered that a breakfast that is higher in protein, where protein and carbohydrates were fairly equal, allowed students to perform significantly better on various cognitive and memory tests (designed to mimic typical work tasks) than after a breakfast that was high in carbs and lower in protein.

Getting your breakfast protein from eggs is not only smart because they provide quality protein but also because research shows that those who start their day with eggs eat less throughout the rest of the day.

Research from St. Louis University (Missouri) found that women who ate eggs, toast and jelly for breakfast reported feeling more full and they ate almost 300 calories less the rest of the day than when they ate a bagel and cream cheese for breakfast.[1] The follow-up study by the same research team confirmed that those eating the egg breakfast lost significantly more body fat than those eating the bagel breakfast.[2] This is likely due to the protein from the eggs, as higher protein meals have been found by researchers at University College London to lead to a greater increase in a hormone known as peptide YY (PYY) that signals the brain to decrease hunger and increase satiety by three times more than after eating a higher-carb meal.[3]

> ## Glucose:
> A term for blood sugar. Glucose is the major sugar the body uses for fuel. The majority of the carbohydrates that we eat are broken down into glucose for our bodies to use as fuel.

Protein sources emphasized on the *PrayFit* diet are low-to-moderate fat proteins such as from poultry, seafood, lean cuts of beef, eggs and low-fat dairy products.

PrayFit Carbs

While many diet experts focus on carbohydrates as the major foundation of their recommended diets—they are either emphasized or demonized—carbs play second fiddle to protein in the *PrayFit* diet. The reason is not only due to all of the benefits of protein discussed above, but to the fact that carbohydrates are a nonessential macronutrient. That means your body does not require carbohydrates to function. This is because your body can make glucose out of amino acids when necessary. Therefore, the *PrayFit* diet does not put much emphasis on carbohydrates, but only places emphasis on choosing certain types of carbohydrates.

The *PrayFit* diet emphasizes slow-digesting carbohydrates, or those with a low glycemic index. The slower the food is digested and absorbed, the lower the glycemic index. Research from Loughborough University found that when athletes ate low GI carbohydrates at breakfast and lunch, they had lower insulin and glucose levels and burned more fat throughout the day than when they consumed high GI carbohydrates.[4]

One low glycemic food emphasized on the *PrayFit* diet is oatmeal. Not only will it help maintain steady insulin and glucose, as well as burn more fat, but research also shows that it helps to lower cholesterol levels, blood pressure and blood glucose levels. In fact, the benefits of oatmeal are so powerful that oatmeal consumption is promoted by the American Dietetic Association (ADA) and the American Heart Association (AHA); and the U.S. Food and Drug administration (FDA) has approved the claims that oats aid cholesterol reduction.

Another whole-grain low-GI food emphasized on the *PrayFit* diet is Ezekiel 4:9 bread. It is named for the passage in the Bible that advises taking grains and legumes, mixing them together and making bread that contains no flour but is instead a mix of organic sprouted whole grains, like wheat, millet, spelt and barley, and legumes like lentils and soybeans. This makes the bread not only a source of very low GI carbs, but also a good source of complete protein.

Fruit is also emphasized on the *PrayFit* diet. Few people realize that most fruits are actually very low GI carbohydrates, due to the fructose and fiber they contain. Eating a wide variety of fruits is a vital part of the *PrayFit* nutritional plan because that will provide a wide range of phytonutrients, such as antioxidants, which are critical for promoting health and longevity, as well as preventing many diseases. Fruits such as berries are particularly emphasized, due to their higher content of antioxidants. So are grapefruit and grapefruit juice, as research from Scripps Clinic in San Diego shows that regularly eating grapefruit, or drinking grapefruit juice, can lead to significant weight loss—even without dieting.[5]

> **Glycemic Index:** A method to measure the rate at which carbohydrates are digested and absorbed by the body.

One specific strategy that the *PrayFit* diet implements is the gradual lowering of carbohydrate intake as the day progresses. With dinner and with your late-night snack, it is suggested that you focus on protein, low-carbohydrate and high-fiber vegetables and healthy fats. The reason for this is that as the day begins to close, most people become significantly less active than they were during the day—they are winding down and preparing for rest; therefore, they require fewer calories during this period and less energy from carbohydrates.

Also, toward the end of the day insulin sensitivity decreases. This means that it takes more insulin to encourage the uptake of glucose (from dietary carbohydrates) into cells. This is bad for two main reasons. For one, the greater insulin required can lead to greater fat storage. Second, the greater release of insulin can lead to type 2 diabetes over time. In addition, research shows that when subjects ate a carbohydrate-rich meal several hours before bedtime they had higher body temperature and faster heart rates than when they consumed the high carbohydrate meal earlier in the day. These factors can negatively affect sleep. Reducing carbohydrate intake later in the day is wise for reducing body fat, maintaining health and helping you sleep better at night.

PrayFit Fats

Fat used to be considered the ultimate dietary no-no. Years of research now shows that fats, even the saturated variety, are not the villainous, body-ruining scourge they once were thought to be.

The Malmo Diet and Cancer Study reported that individuals receiving more than 30 percent of their total daily energy from fat and more than 10 percent from saturated fat did not have increased mortality.[6] Research from Loma Linda University (California) concluded that a higher-fat diet consisting of 39 percent fat (mostly from healthy fats such as almonds) and 32 percent carbohydrates resulted in a 56 percent greater fat loss than a diet composed of 53 percent carbs and only 18 percent fat.[7]

The *PrayFit* dietary plan emphasizes healthy monounsaturated and polyunsaturated fat sources such as nuts, seeds, olives and olive oil, and avocadoes and essential omega-3 fatty acid sources, such as salmon, trout, herring, as well as flaxseeds and walnuts. These healthy fats can help fend off diseases and even promote athletic performance.

The Skinny On Fat:

Saturated fats are fatty acids that are saturated with hydrogen. This type of fat is associated with a higher risk of cardiovascular disease.

Unsaturated fats are fatty acids that are not saturated with hydrogen atoms, meaning that a hydrogen atom has been replaced with a double bond.

Monounsaturated fats have one hydrogen atom missing and can help to lower cholesterol levels and aid fat loss. Polyunsaturated fats have more than one hydrogen atom missing. One type of polyunsaturated fat, omega-3 fat, provides numerous health benefits such as enhanced fat loss, better heart health and even reduced risk of certain cancers.

Trans fats are unsaturated fats that have been artificially saturated with hydrogen atoms. Trans fats should be avoided at all costs, as they have been shown to increase fat gain and promote cardiovascular disease, diabetes and certain cancers.

Mono- and polyunsaturated fats help to lower total blood cholesterol and triglycerides and raise HDL cholesterol (the good cholesterol) levels in the blood. These fats, particularly the omega-3 polyunsaturated fats, also help prevent chronic inflammatory-related diseases such as cardiovascular disease. In addition, they may improve insulin sensitivity and blood pressure, reducing the risk of diabetes and hypertension, as well as help to prevent certain cancers. Mono- and polyunsaturated fats also are readily burned for fuel to provide you more energy throughout the day, and research shows that the omega-3 fats can actually promote fat loss.

The only fat that the *PrayFit* diet condemns is trans fat. Trans fats promote heart disease, diabetes, certain cancers and obesity. They also raise LDL cholesterol (the bad cholesterol) levels, C-reactive protein and triglycerides. In addition, trans fats lower HDL cholesterol levels and may encourage muscle breakdown. Combined, all of these factors should make you rethink food choices that are higher in trans fats. (Hint: Many of your favorite drive-thru foods contain trans fats.)

PrayFit Nutrition Principles

Eat more often. Research shows that eating smaller, more frequent meals throughout the day supports a higher metabolic rate and significantly decreases hunger better than eating fewer bigger meals. This lack of hunger makes it easy to maintain the *PrayFit* diet plan and adopt it as a lifestyle.

Modest caloric intake. While this may seem to run contrary to the "eat all day long" principle above, it doesn't. Despite the frequency of eating, you still only consume about 1,800 calories each day with the *PrayFit* nutrition plan.

Decreased carb consumption at night. Cutting your consumption of carbs as the day goes on—after lunch is a good time to start your decline—will help you get better sleep and decrease the likelihood that you will store body fat from a late, high-carb meal.

Balance and simplicity. This plan provides practical, easily applicable dietary guidelines for anyone with almost any goal. Whether you wish to lose weight, feel better, be healthier, get fitter, have more energy or all of the above, the *PrayFit* diet can help you reach your goals by providing you a well-balanced diet that is equal in calories from protein, carbohydrates and fat.

Options. Unlike some rigid diets, *PrayFit* allows you options—so long as you follow the suggested guidelines, of course. Some alternative meals are presented on pages 219-224.

A community table. Since what you eat can go a long way toward determining how much—or how little—your body will change over the next few weeks, it's important to take advantage of every resource available to you. Send us a question at prayfit.com or share your dietary progress (or recipes) with other readers at prayfit.com/forums.

Notes

1. J. S. Vander Wal, et al., "Short-term Effect of Eggs on Satiety in Overweight and Obese Subjects," *Journal of the American College of Nutrition*, December 2005, vol. 24, no. 6, pp. 510-515.

2. Ibid.

3. R. L. Batterham, et al., "Critical Role for Peptide YY in Protein-mediated Satiation and Body-weight Regulation," *Cell Metabolism*, 2006, vol. 4, no. 3, pp. 223-233.

4. E. Stevenson, et al., "The Influence of the Glycaemic Index of Breakfast and Lunch on Substrate Utilisation During the Postprandial Periods and Subsequent Exercise, *British Journal of Nutrition,* 2005, vol. 93, no. 6, pp. 885-893.

5. K. Fujioka, et al., "The Effects of Grapefruit on Weight and Insulin Resistance: Relationship to the Metabolic Syndrome," *Journal of Medicinal Food*, Spring 2006, vol. 9, no. 1, pp. 49-54.

6. M. Leosdottir, et al., "Dietary Fat Intake and Early Mortality Patterns—Data from The Malmo Diet and Cancer Study," Journal of Internal Medicine, August 2005, vol. 258, no. 2, pp. 153-165.

7. M. A. Wien, et al., "Almonds vs. Complex Carbohydrates in a Weight Reduction Program," *International Journal of Obesity and Related Metabolic Disorders*, November 2003, vol. 11, pp. 1365-1372.

PrayFit: The Exercises

Proper execution of the exercises in the 28-day *PrayFit* program will not only ensure consistent progress but will also help you avoid injury. Follow these easy steps to get the most out of each of the 10 movements in the *PrayFit* program. (For video demonstrations of these exercises and others, visit www.prayfit.com/fitness.)

Upper Body Exercises

Standard Push-Up or Modified Push-Up on Knees
Focus: Chest, shoulders, back, abs

Get into a push-up position with your body in a straight line, feet together, hands wider than shoulder width apart and your eyes focused on the floor. Press yourself up to full arm extension, keeping your abs tight and back straight. Squeeze your arms and chest at the top, then lower yourself to the start and repeat. Don't bounce your chest off the floor, but rather start each rep when your chest reaches a point an inch or so away from the floor.

Incline Push-Up
Focus: Lower chest, shoulders, back, abs

Find a wall, a sturdy end of a couch or a flat bench and place your hands against it wider than shoulder width apart. With your feet stable a couple of feet behind you, press until your arms are fully extended. Flex and squeeze your chest, shoulders and arms at the top, then slowly lower yourself to the start. When your chest reaches an inch or so away from the stable platform, press yourself up again and repeat.

Decline Push-Up
Focus: Upper chest, shoulders, back, abs

Get into a push-up position with your feet elevated on a stool or bench or couch. Place your hands wider than shoulder width apart and your eyes focused on the floor. Press yourself up to full arm extension, keeping your abs tight and back straight. Squeeze your arms and chest at the top, then lower yourself to the start. When your face reaches an inch or so away from the floor, explode back up to the fully extended position.

> ## Firm Believer:
> By slightly altering the angle on your push-ups, you can make subtle changes to how the muscles of the chest are trained. This four-week program includes the three most common angles to help give your chest training the greatest variety possible.

Lower Body Exercises

Bodyweight Squat
Focus: Legs, glutes, hamstrings, lower back

Stand with your feet about shoulder width apart, a light bend in your knees and your toes turned out slightly. Keeping your head neutral, abs tight and torso erect, bend at the knees and hips to slowly lower your body as if you were going to sit down in a chair. Pause when your legs reach a 90-degree angle, then forcefully drive through your heels, extending at your hips and knees until you arrive at the standing position.

Lunge
Focus: Legs, glutes, hamstrings, lower back

Stand with your feet together, abs tight and eyes focused forward. Step forward with one foot. Bend both knees to lower yourself, making sure your front knee doesn't pass your toes on your front foot. Stop just short of your rear knee touching the floor and reverse directions, driving through the heel of your forward foot to return to the start. Alternate legs for reps.

Abdominal Exercises

Crunch
Focus: Upper abs

Lie face-up on the floor with your hands cupped gently behind your head (do not pull on your neck). Keeping your knees bent and with your feet flat on the floor, crunch your upper body up until your shoulder blades are off the floor. Squeeze your abs, then lower yourself back to the start and repeat.

Reverse Crunch
Focus: Lower abs

Lie face-up on the floor with your hands extended at your sides, your feet up and knees bent at a 90-degree angle. Your thighs should be perpendicular to the floor. Slowly bring your knees toward your chest, lifting your hips and glutes off the ground, and try to maintain the bend in your knees throughout the movement. Return under control.

Firm Believer:

Whether you're a man or a woman, you need to take your lower-body training seriously. Pouring as much intensity into these exercises as possible is one of the biggest favors you can do for your physique. Your legs contain some of the largest muscles in your body. Working them hard ensures a greater total caloric burn and more significant change in overall body composition.

Double Crunch
Focus: Upper abs, lower abs

Lie down on the floor with your legs straight, feet together. Place your hands gently behind your head and raise your feet off the floor roughly six inches. Crunch your upper body off the floor while simultaneously bringing your knees toward your torso, so that your upper body meets your lower body in the middle. Squeeze and return to the start, allowing your legs to remain above the floor throughout.

Firm Believer:

Incorporating power training into your workouts enhances your overall athleticism and helps you build more muscle in the long run. Plus, it provides a new challenge, which is a key component of achieving long-term change with your physique.

Power Exercises

Jump Squat
Focus: Legs, glutes, hamstrings, lower back, calves

Stand with both hands directly in front of you, knees slightly bent with roughly a shoulder width stance. Keeping your chest up and back flat, squat down until your thighs approach parallel with the floor, then explode upward as high as possible, allowing your feet to leave the floor. Land on soft feet with your knees bent, and repeat immediately.

Power Push-Up
Focus: Lower chest, shoulders, back, abs

Get into a push-up position with your body in a straight line, feet together, hands wider than shoulder width apart and your eyes focused on the floor. Explode yourself up to full arm extension, allowing your hands to leave the floor. Catch yourself with your hands on the floor and decelerate yourself to the start, then repeat. Don't bounce your chest off the floor, but rather start each rep when your chest reaches an inch or so away from it.

PrayFit: Menu Options

The meal component of *PrayFit* is vitally important to your progress. These 28 to 56 days are loosely prescriptive. We provide a baseline example in "PrayFit: Eating in Balance" on pages 205-213, but some healthy variety will keep you from getting bored.

In this section we present four options for the day's three main meals and four options for snack times. Included are the calorie counts and macronutrient breakdowns for each meal. Keeping to these choices will fuel your workouts and recovery in the right way, helping you make significant, lasting change in the way you look, feel and perform.

When you add all of these options to the standard *PrayFit* menu and the three tasty recipes we present each week, you'll have a wide array of food combinations from which to choose each day.

Breakfast

Your first meal of the day sets the tone for the rest of your day. Upon waking, it's important to call a definitive halt to the fast your body has endured during sleep. This is accomplished with a generous dose of protein, which will provide your muscles with much-needed amino acids for energy and recovery, a modest portion of healthy carbohydrates to refuel depleted stores, and a sprinkle of healthy fats to aid in digestion and other bodily functions.

Lunch

Lunch is an important bridge between your morning meal and dinner, regardless of when you work out. If you work out in the morning, lunch provides triage to muscles that are already knee-deep in the recovery process. If you work out in the evening, it's important to secure the right energy for the road ahead. And if you're not working out today, you still need to make sure you have a nutritious lunch to help keep energy levels and focus in check throughout the afternoon. In other words, it's not a throwaway meal. You'll notice that the carb counts are fairly generous in these options. Remember, the *PrayFit* plan has you reducing carbs as the day goes on, and lunch constitutes the start of that decline.

Dinner

How you finish your day is as important as how you start it. If you go completely off the nutritional radar for dinner, that can lead to further slip-ups the next day. Eating right will put your body in an excellent position to recover while you sleep. These high-protein dishes provide a gradual release of amino acids to your muscles throughout the night, keeping your progress moving, even while you're not.

Snacks

On *PrayFit*, you'll be taking a departure from the traditional "three squares a day" philosophy. Feeding your body correctly throughout the day—not only at the three major meals—is the key to keeping your energy up and your sanity in check. These between-meal snacks toss some kindling on your metabolic fire, keeping it burning hotter and longer. Plus, it helps you avoid feeling deprived of food, which means you won't feel the need to gorge at any meals.

For a sample week of the PrayFit diet, see the next section.

Breakfast

Breakfast	Calories	Protein (g)	Carbs (g)	Fat (g)
Option 1: 1 cup cooked oatmeal ½ cup fresh berries 1 tbsp chopped walnuts 2 slices cooked turkey bacon	296	20	37	8
Option 2: 1 egg plus 3 egg whites, scrambled 3 slices tomato 1 Ezekiel 4:9 tortilla 6 fl oz grapefruit juice	358	25	45	9
Option 3: 1 cup low-fat cottage cheese ¾ cup chopped pineapple 2 tbsp ground flaxseed 6 fl oz grapefruit juice	370	32	43	8

Option 4:
1 slice Ezekiel 4:9 bread
1 tbsp natural peanut
    butter
6 oz nonfat plain Greek
    yogurt
1 peach, chopped
	336	24	40	9

Lunch

Lunch	Calories	Protein (g)	Carbs (g)	Fat (g)
Option 1: 3 cups baby spinach ½ cup chopped tomato ½ cup chickpeas 4 oz grilled chicken breast 1 tsp olive oil + 1 tbsp balsamic vinegar	432	46	39	10
Option 2: 4 oz turkey deli meat 1 slice low-fat cheddar cheese 2 tbsp salsa 2 slices Ezekiel 4:9 bread	338	30	37	7
Option 3: 4 oz broiled or grilled salmon ½ cup cooked brown rice ¼ cup black beans 1 cup steamed broccoli	426	41	44	10
Option 4: 4 oz grilled chicken breast 1 baked sweet potato 2 cups mixed greens 1 tbsp light vinaigrette salad dressing	421	40	42	9

Dinner

Dinner	Calories	Protein (g)	Carbs (g)	Fat (g)
Option 1: 4 oz grilled or broiled flank steak 1 ½ cups roasted broccoli 2 cups mixed greens 1 tbsp olive oil + 1 tbsp vinegar	451	39	23	24
Option 2: 4 oz baked salmon or tuna 1 cup steamed spinach 1 cup sliced cucumber 1 cup chopped tomato 1 ½ oz feta cheese, crumbled 2 tsp olive oil	439	40	19	24
Option 3: 4 oz cooked turkey burger 1 ½ cups steamed green beans 3 tbsp slivered almonds 2 tbsp light vinaigrette salad dressing	435	30	22	27
Option 4: 1 cup minestrone soup with 2 tbsp grated Parmesan cheese 4 oz roasted chicken breast 1 ½ cups steamed asparagus with 1 tbsp olive oil	510	49	30	23

Snacks

Snacks	Calories	Protein (g)	Carbs (g)	Fat (g)
Option 1: 1 cup grapes 1 part-skim mozzarella string cheese 2 oz turkey deli meat	202	15	19	8
Option 2: $1/_3$ cup low-fat cottage cheese $1/_3$ cup fresh berries 7 almonds	130	12	11	5
Option 3: 5 medium baby carrots 1 cup steamed edamame with salt	198	15	17	8
Option 4: $1/_3$ cup nonfat Greek yogurt $1/_3$ cup fresh berries 1 tbsp walnuts	130	12	10	5

PrayFit:
Sample Menu Week

Day 1

Breakfast	Calories	Protein (g)	Carbs (g)	Fat (g)
1 whole large egg	74	6	0	5
3 large egg whites	51	12	0	0
1 slice low-fat American cheese	38	5	1	1
½ cup dry oatmeal	145	6	25	2
6 oz. grapefruit juice	72	1	17	0

Scramble eggs and add cheese. Prepare oatmeal as directed on package; add artificial sweetener if desired.

Late-morning snack	Calories	Protein (g)	Carbs (g)	Fat (g)
1 cup chicken noodle soup	5	6	9	2
½ cup low-fat cottage cheese	82	14	3	1
½ cup sliced pineapple	40	1	10	0

Mix pineapple in cottage cheese and eat—can use ½ cup of any kind of sliced fruit as well, or blueberries or other berries instead.

Lunch	Calories	Protein (g)	Carbs (g)	Fat (g)
4 oz. turkey deli meat	104	22	2	0
1 slice low-fat American cheese	38	5	1	1
2 slices Ezekiel 4:9 bread	160	8	30	1
1 tbsp. fat-free mayonnaise	11	0	2	0

Make sandwich with ingredients; can also use 4 oz. fat-free ham instead; can use any type of low-fat cheese; can use mustard instead of mayo.

Mid-day snack	Calories	Protein (g)	Carbs (g)	Fat (g)
8 oz. plain low-fat yogurt	143	12	16	4
½ cup blueberries	42	1	11	0

Mix berries in yogurt and eat; can also use other types of berries or sliced fruit instead.

Dinner	Calories	Protein (g)	Carbs (g)	Fat (g)
6 oz. salmon	312	34	0	18
1 cup chopped broccoli	31	3	6	0
2 cups mixed green salad	44	3	8	0
2 tbsp salad dressing (olive oil and vinegar)	144	0	0	16

Bake or broil salmon with any herbs or spices desired—can also eat same amount of baked or broiled tilapia, snapper, cod or similar fish, or chicken or turkey breast, or once per week substitute same amount of lean beef such as top sirloin or flank steak. Steam or boil broccoli—can also use 1 cup of other veggies such as cauliflower, green beans, asparagus, Brussels sprouts, or sliced zucchini instead.

Nighttime snack	Calories	Protein (g)	Carbs (g)	Fat (g)
1 oz. mixed nuts	168	5	7	15

Day 1 TOTALS	Calories	Protein (g)	Carbs (g)	Fat (g)
	1,775	144	148	66
Percent of total calories	—	33%	33%	33%
Calories or grams/pound body weight*	12 cal.	1.0 gram	1.0 gram	0.5 gram

*Though the reference weight here is 150 pounds, this applies for a person weighing 130 to 250 pounds. The recommendations hold because of how it will affect a person at the higher end of that scale who is perhaps carrying more body fat. For more precise guidelines for your body weight, visit prayfit.com.

Day 2

Breakfast	Calories	Protein (g)	Carbs (g)	Fat (g)
1 cup cooked oatmeal	147	6	25	2
½ cup fresh berries	32	1	7	0
7 walnuts, chopped	92	2	2	9
3 slices extra-lean turkey bacon	60	9	0	2

Add walnuts and berries to oatmeal.

Late-morning snack	Calories	Protein (g)	Carbs (g)	Fat (g)
1½ cups grapes	93	2	24	0
2 sticks light mozzarella string cheese	100	12	2	6

Lunch	Calories	Protein (g)	Carbs (g)	Fat (g)
3 cups baby spinach	21	3	3	0
½ cup chopped tomato	16	1	3	0
½ cup chickpeas	143	6	27	2
4 oz. grilled chicken breast, sliced	124	28	0	1
1 tsp. olive oil	40	0	0	5
1 tbsp. balsamic vinegar	0	0	0	0

Mix all ingredients together to make salad, and top with olive oil and vinegar.

Midday snack	Calories	Protein (g)	Carbs (g)	Fat (g)
1 cup steamed soybeans (edamame)	254	22	20	12

Dinner	Calories	Protein (g)	Carbs (g)	Fat (g)
4 oz. grilled or broiled flank steak	174	24	0	8
1½ cups chopped broccoli, roasted	46	5	9	0
2 cups mixed greens	44	3	8	0
1 tbsp. olive oil	119	0	0	14
1 tbsp. balsamic vinegar	0	0	0	0

Nighttime snack	Calories	Protein (g)	Carbs (g)	Fat (g)
2 hardboiled eggs	148	12	0	10

Day 2 TOTALS	Calories	Protein (g)	Carbs (g)	Fat (g)
	1,653	163	130	71
Percent of total calories	—1	33%	31%	36%
Calories or grams/pound body weight*	11 cal.	1.0 gram	1.0 gram	0.5 gram

*Though the reference weight here is 150 pounds, this applies for a person weighing 130 to 250 pounds. The recommendations hold because of how it will affect a person at the higher end of that scale who is perhaps carrying more body fat. For more precise guidelines for your body weight, visit prayfit.com.

Day 3

Breakfast	Calories	Protein (g)	Carbs (g)	Fat (g)
1 Ezekiel 4:9 tortilla	150	6	24	4
1 large whole egg	74	6	0	5
3 egg whites	51	12	0	0
1 slice tomato	5	0	1	0
8 oz. grapefruit juice	96	1	23	0

Scramble eggs, place on tortilla, add tomato slices and roll it.

Late-morning snack	Calories	Protein (g)	Carbs (g)	Fat (g)
2 medium stalks of celery	12	0	2	0
2 tbsp. peanut butter	188	8	6	18

Chop celery into 4-inch pieces and fill center with peanut butter.

Lunch	Calories	Protein (g)	Carbs (g)	Fat (g)
4 oz. turkey deli meat	104	22	2	0
2 slices Ezekiel 4:9 bread	160	8	30	2
2 tbsp. salsa	8	0	2	0

Midday snack	Calories	Protein (g)	Carbs (g)	Fat (g)
1 large apple	110	0	30	0
2 oz. fat-free cheese (Swiss, cheddar, etc.)	80	16	2	0

Dinner	Calories	Protein (g)	Carbs (g)	Fat (g)
6 oz. grilled or broiled salmon	312	34	0	18
1 cup sautéed spinach	7	1	1	0
1 medium cucumber, sliced	24	1	4	0
1 cup chopped tomato	32	2	7	0
1 oz. fat-free feta	35	7	1	0
1 tbsp. olive oil	119	0	0	14

Nighttime snack	Calories	Protein (g)	Carbs (g)	Fat (g)
1 cup low-fat cottage cheese	163	28	6	2
2 tbsp. roasted flaxseeds	90	3	4	7

Day 3 TOTALS	Calories	Protein (g)	Carbs (g)	Fat (g)
	1,820	155	145	70
Percent of total calories	—	34%	32%	34%
Calories or grams/pound body weight*	12 cal.	1.0 gram	1.0 gram	0.5 gram

*Though the reference weight here is 150 pounds, this applies for a person weighing 130 to 250 pounds. The recommendations hold because of how it will affect a person at the higher end of that scale who is perhaps carrying more body fat. For more precise guidelines for your body weight, visit prayfit.com.

Day 4

Breakfast	Calories	Protein (g)	Carbs (g)	Fat (g)
1 cup low-fat cottage cheese	163	28	6	2
1 cup sliced pineapple	79	1	20	0
2 tbsp. roasted flax seeds	90	3	4	7
8 oz. grapefruit juice	96	1	23	0

Late-morning snack	Calories	Protein (g)	Carbs (g)	Fat (g)
1 cup chicken noodle soup	76	6	9	2
½ cup low-fat cottage cheese	82	14	3	1
½ cup sliced pineapple	40	1	10	0

Lunch	Calories	Protein (g)	Carbs (g)	Fat (g)
3 oz. grilled or broiled salmon	156	17	0	9
½ cup brown rice, cooked	109	3	23	1
½ cup black beans	113	8	20	1
1 cup chopped broccoli, steamed	31	3	6	0

Midday snack	Calories	Protein (g)	Carbs (g)	Fat (g)
1 cup boiled soybeans (edamame)	254	22	20	12

Dinner	Calories	Protein (g)	Carbs (g)	Fat (g)
4 oz. turkey burger	140	16	0	8
1 cup green beans	36	2	8	0
2 tbsp. sliced almonds	90	4	3	8
1 tbsp. olive oil	119	0	0	14
1 tbsp. balsamic vinegar	0	0	0	0

Add almonds, olive oil and vinegar to green beans.

Nighttime snack	Calories	Protein (g)	Carbs (g)	Fat (g)
1 oz. beef jerky	60	9	3	1

Day 4 TOTALS	Calories	Protein (g)	Carbs (g)	Fat (g)
	1,734	138	158	66
Percent of total calories	—	32%	34%	34%
Calories or grams/pound body weight*	12 cal.	1.0 gram	1.0 gram	0.5 gram

*Though the reference weight here is 150 pounds, this applies for a person weighing 130 to 250 pounds. The recommendations hold because of how it will affect a person at the higher end of that scale who is perhaps carrying more body fat. For more precise guidelines for your body weight, visit prayfit.com.

Day 5

Breakfast	Calories	Protein (g)	Carbs (g)	Fat (g)
1 slice Ezekiel 4:9 bread	80	4	15	1
1 tbsp. peanut butter	94	4	3	8
1 cup reduced fat Greek yogurt	150	19	9	5
1 tbsp. honey	64	0	17	0

Spread peanut butter on bread. Mix honey in yogurt.

Late-morning snack	Calories	Protein (g)	Carbs (g)	Fat (g)
1½ cups grapes	93	2	24	0
2 sticks light mozzarella string cheese	100	12	2	6

Lunch	Calories	Protein (g)	Carbs (g)	Fat (g)
4 oz. chicken breast	124	28	0	1
1 medium sweet potato	103	2	24	0
2 cups mixed greens	44	3	8	0
1 tbsp. olive oil	119	0	0	14
1 tbsp. balsamic vinegar	0	0	0	0

Midday snack	Calories	Protein (g)	Carbs (g)	Fat (g)
1 cup low-fat cottage cheese	163	28	6	2
1 cup blueberries	83	1	21	0

Dinner	Calories	Protein (g)	Carbs (g)	Fat (g)
1 cup minestrone soup	82	4	11	3
2 tbsp. grated Parmesan cheese	25	2	0	2
4 oz. chicken breast	124	28	0	1
1 cup asparagus	27	3	5	0
1 tbsp. olive oil	119	0	0	14

Nighttime snack	Calories	Protein (g)	Carbs (g)	Fat (g)
2 hardboiled eggs	148	12	0	10

Day 5 TOTALS	Calories	Protein (g)	Carbs (g)	Fat (g)
	1,742	152	145	67
Percent of total calories	—	34%	32%	34%
Calories or grams/pound body weight*	1.0 gram	1.0gram	1.0 gram	0.5 gram

*Though the reference weight here is 150 pounds, this applies for a person weighing 130 to 250 pounds. The recommendations hold because of how it will affect a person at the higher end of that scale who is perhaps carrying more body fat. For more precise guidelines for your body weight, visit prayfit.com.

Day 6

Breakfast	Calories	Protein (g)	Carbs (g)	Fat (g)
1 medium sweet potato, chopped	103	2	24	0
½ medium onion, diced	23	1	6	0
1 tbsp. olive oil	119	0	0	14
1 whole large egg	74	6	0	5
3 egg whites, large	51	12	0	0

Fry sweet potato and onion in a pan coated with olive oil to make sweet potato home fries. Scramble eggs and cook in a nonstick cooking pan.

Late-morning snack	Calories	Protein (g)	Carbs (g)	Fat (g)
1 cup reduced-fat Greek yogurt	150	19	9	5
1 tbsp. honey	64	0	17	0
¼ cup shelled sunflower seeds	170	7	5	15

Mix honey and seeds in yogurt.

Lunch	Calories	Protein (g)	Carbs (g)	Fat (g)
1 (5 oz.) can chunk light tuna in water	125	28	0	1
1 cup whole-wheat pasta	174	7	37	1
½ medium onion, diced	23	1	6	0
1 medium celery stalk, diced	6	0	1	0
4 large black olives, diced	20	0	1	2
1 tbsp. light mayonnaise	50	0	1	5
1 tbsp. olive oil	119	0	0	14
1 tsp. red wine vinegar	0	0	0	0

Cook pasta and chill in refrigerator. Add all ingredients to pasta and mix to make a Mediterranean pasta salad.

Midday snack	Calories	Protein (g)	Carbs (g)	Fat (g)
1 cup chicken noodle soup	76	6	9	2
½ cup low-fat cottage cheese	82	14	3	1
½ cup sliced pineapple	40	1	10	0

Mix pineapple in cottage cheese.

Dinner	Calories	Protein (g)	Carbs (g)	Fat (g)
6 oz. top sirloin steak	216	36	0	6
1 cup cooked spaghetti squash	42	1	10	0
1 tsp. olive oil	40	0	0	5

Add olive oil to squash and salt and pepper to taste.

Nighttime snack	Calories	Protein (g)	Carbs (g)	Fat (g)
½ cup low-fat cottage cheese	81	14	3	1

Day 6 TOTALS	Calories	Protein (g)	Carbs (g)	Fat (g)
	1,848	155	142	77
Percent of total calories	—	33%	31%	36%
Calories or grams/pound body weight*	12 cal.	1.0 gram	1.0 gram	0.5 gram

*Though the reference weight here is 150 pounds, this applies for a person weighing 130 to 250 pounds. The recommendations hold because of how it will affect a person at the higher end of that scale who is perhaps carrying more body fat. For more precise guidelines for your body weight, visit prayfit.com.

Day 7

Breakfast	Calories	Protein (g)	Carbs (g)	Fat (g)
1 large egg	74	6	0	5
1 egg white	17	4	0	0
1 slice reduced-fat cheese	90	8	1	6
3 slices extra lean turkey bacon	60	9	0	2
1 Ezekiel English muffin	160	8	30	1

Fry eggs in skillet. Fry bacon in separate skillet. Toast muffin. Place eggs on one side of muffin, add cheese, then bacon and top with other side of muffin to make breakfast muffin.

Late-morning snack	Calories	Protein (g)	Carbs (g)	Fat (g)
1 large apple	110	0	30	0
2 oz. fat-free cheese	80	16	2	0

Lunch	Calories	Protein (g)	Carbs (g)	Fat (g)
2 slices Ezekiel 4:9 bread	160	8	30	2
1 slice reduced-fat cheese	90	8	1	6
1 slice low-fat ham	31	5	1	1
2 cups mixed greens	44	3	8	0
1 tbsp. olive oil	119	2	0	14
1 tbsp. balsamic vinegar	0	0	0	0

Place ham and cheese on bread to make sandwich, and cook in a skillet to make a ham and cheese melt.

Midday snack	Calories	Protein (g)	Carbs (g)	Fat (g)
8 oz. reduced-fat Greek yogurt	150	19	9	5
1 tbsp. honey	64	0	17	0
1 tbsp. peanut butter	94	4	3	8

Mix peanut butter and honey in yogurt.

Dinner	Calories	Protein (g)	Carbs (g)	Fat (g)
2 chicken drumsticks	152	26	0	5
½ medium boiled artichoke	32	2	7	0
1 tbsp. olive oil	119	0	0	14

Sprinkle garlic salt and other desired spices on the chicken and bake at 375° F for 40 minutes in baking dish. Remove skin after cooking. Add salt and pepper to olive oil in small bowl and dip artichoke leaves in oil mix before eating.

Nighttime snack	Calories	Protein (g)	Carbs (g)	Fat (g)
2 oz. beef jerky	120	18	6	2

Day 7 TOTALS	Calories	Protein (g)	Carbs (g)	Fat (g)
	1,766	144	145	71
Percent of total calories	—	33%	33%	34%
Calories or grams/pound body weight*	1.0 gram	1.0 gram	1.0 gram	0.5 gram

*Though the reference weight here is 150 pounds, this applies for a person weighing 130 to 250 pounds. The recommendations hold because of how it will affect a person at the higher end of that scale who is perhaps carrying more body fat. For more precise guidelines for your body weight, visit prayfit.com.

PrayFit Nutrition References

Fischer, K., et al. "Carbohydrate to Protein Ratio in Food and Cognitive Performance in the Morning." *Physiology and Behavior*, March 2002, 75 (3):411-423.

Foster-Powel, K., et al. "International Table of Glycemic Index and Glycemic Load Values: 2002." *American Journal of Clinical Nutrition,* 2002. 76:5-56.

Speechly, D. P., and R. Buffenstein. "Greater Appetite Control Associated with an Increased Frequency of Eating in Lean Males." *Appetite,* 1999. 33(3):285-297.

Stevenson, E., et al. "The Influence of the Glycaemic Index of Breakfast and Lunch on Substrate Utilisation During the Postprandial Periods and Subsequent Exercise." *British Journal of Nutrition,* 2005. 93(6):885-893.

Vander Wal, J. S., et al. "Short-term Effect of Eggs on Satiety in Overweight and Obese Subjects." *Journal of the American College of Nutrition*, December 2005. 24(6):510-515.

Vander Wal, J. S., et al. "Egg Breakfast Enhances Weight Loss." *International Journal of Obesity* (London), October 2008. 32(10):1545-1551.

Gone Are the Days

With the windows rolled down, we'd let our hands pierce the wind as we drove down the highway. Like most brothers, Bubba and I did our share of fighting in the backseat. Of course, being the younger of the two, the fun times usually ended when I started crying. Interestingly, of my life's buried memories, times together as a family—at dinner tables, in living rooms, backyards and backseats—seem to be the first ones to find their way to the surface of recollection.

Speaking of "from those backseats," my brother and I would spot a perfect football field every few miles. Freshly cut grass with trees for goal lines meant fly-by hours for a couple of kids from Texas. As frequently, Dad would have to slow down to let the street baseball game clear a path. Using parked cars and hydrants as bases, I understood well any looks of disdain from huffing kids as we drove along; what were we doing driving through their game for, anyway?

But gone are the days when kids notice open fields, or dads slow down for children playing. Though boys and girls still sit in backseats, their eyes seldom rise to meet anything but their own computer screen or portable electronic game, while iPods drown out any and all conversation.

Over the last few decades, kids and young adults have lost their health, but I'm not going to repeat the plethora of statistics of obesity you've probably already heard or read, although we've chosen a few shocking stats to share throughout this book. To put it mildly, we are great at identifying problems and offering data to support them. We have no problem adding up the sum of how our lack of attention to our kids' health is crippling a generation, if not the entire world. We're smart. We know what's happening, how it's happening and why. Perhaps the only question we haven't really tried to answer is where to begin. Wait . . . strike that. We know where to begin but don't have the courage to do what needs to be done.

It's ridiculous to think that for the first time in history, kids born today have an appreciable chance of not outliving their parents. In other words, if you have a child under the age of five, they'll die before you. Plain as that. You are more likely to bury your kids due to the complications of obesity than they are to bury you from natural causes.

But again, as shocking as that statistic is, you and I turn this page as easy as it would be had we not even read it. I'm not sure why, but perhaps it's because our generation has seen more catastrophes and experienced more disease and famine than any other, and a silent yet efficient killer like obesity just doesn't have enough shock for us to give it value.

We at PrayFit applaud the efforts of government to help clean up food choices in schools, and we love programming that's attacking the idea of cleaner eating. But it's not about food alone. In fact, as kids, we didn't eat all that great growing up. Well, we certainly finished what was on our plates, but we had fun and worked it all off without knowing it. And that's the difference. Sure, kids need more fruits and vegetables and less fast food, but unless they move their bodies (and have fun doing it without a prescription to "play at least an hour a day"), a healthy child in America will soon be a thing of the past. And an open field will forever take a backseat to a good text message and a Happy Meal.

It's Time to Lead

A Note to Pastors and Other Leaders

Jimmy Page
Fellowship of Christian Athletes

I recently had an opportunity to present to two different groups of leaders about the same topic. The first group of leaders were coaches; the second were full-time ministry leaders. What these two groups had in common was an enormous platform to influence others.

It's been said that one coach will impact more young people in one year than the average person will in a lifetime. And leaders in full-time vocational ministry bring a message of life transformation week in and week out. As a father, a coach and a full-time ministry guy, I can relate to both groups in a personal way.

Interestingly enough, the majority of both groups were in relatively poor health—overweight, tired, stressed and inactive. They were worn out, but somehow most didn't make the connection between their lifestyle choices and their effectiveness in their jobs. They were making poor choices with food even though they knew the right choices to make. Most had not consistently invested in their physical health, and it showed.

One of my core life principles is that I won't preach what I don't practice. Now that doesn't mean that I have to be perfect in a given area, but I do need to be striving and making progress in an area before I will pass on wisdom to others. I really believe that it's a matter of integrity. Don't tell others what they should do if you aren't willing to do it yourself.

One of the biggest gaps I've seen develop over the last 20 years is the gap between knowing and doing, especially in the area of personal health. In America, we have access to more credible information about how to eat and exercise for good health than at any other time in history. We know that we should eat an abundance of fruits and vegetables. We know that we should eat whole grains, nuts, beans and seeds. We know that we should go easy on red meat, but eat fish, lean turkey and chicken instead. We know that we should drink water as our primary source of fluids and avoid sodas, juices and anything with high fructose corn syrup. We know that fried foods are bad and that sugary drinks and desserts like ice cream, cookies and cakes will destroy our health and athletic performance. Knowing is the easy part; it's doing that trips us up. And we've become masterful at the art of making excuses.

But perhaps the biggest gap that I've witnessed is in the leadership of the church. We lead on every moral issue of the day—but we fail to lead with respect to personal health. We challenge others to live a life of excellence in every area of life except their health. We map out biblical principles as they relate to our relationships, the workplace, parenting, attitudes, the way we think, and marriage. We raise all the big moral dilemmas and take on the tough issues of pornography, infidelity, abortion and even politics! But the issue of health is like the third rail—we don't touch it. We fail to lead. So the obvious next question is "Why?"

I think there are many reasons, but the first one is simple: As leaders, we can't give away what we don't have. And let's face it—many of us are simply not good stewards of our own health. If you look at church leadership today, we look a lot like everybody else. In fact, some studies indicate that the church and specifically church leadership is in worse shape than the rest of the country. We're out of shape. We're obese. So it's almost impossible to bring the message of being a good steward of your health to the church because the message doesn't ring true. It would be like saying, "Do as I say, not as I do." The gap between what we say and what we do would be obvious, so we don't touch the topic.

Second, we're afraid to offend anyone. It's personal, and nobody can hide. Poor health usually shows up on the outside. If I'm significantly overweight, or regularly overeating, or making poor choices with food, or not exercising, it doesn't take long for the result of my actions to show up on the outside. We can hide from almost every other sin. A pastor could preach on particular sins and no one else would know if he is struggling in that area. We've gotten good at putting on the mask in public. But it's hard to cover up our physical health. So instead of leading, we avoid the topic entirely.

But I believe it's time for the church to take the lead. Church leaders first need to take their own health seriously as an act of obedience and good stewardship. We must "purify ourselves from everything that contaminates body and spirit" (2 Cor. 7:1). Then we need to lead those we influence on the path to better health. We are all called to "offer [our] bodies as living sacrifices, holy and pleasing to God" (Rom. 12:1). When Jesus was asked what the greatest command was, He responded, "Love the Lord your God with all your heart and with all your soul and with all your mind and with all your strength. The second is this: 'Love your neighbor as yourself'" (Mark 12:30-31). Heart, soul, mind and body—that about covers it.

When we're healthy, we have so much more energy for the journey. Our mood is better, we're more positive and optimistic, and we have more endurance for the important things of life.

It's time to get our house in order and lead the charge toward a life of abundant health and life. So if you're a leader or in a position of influence, start taking your own steps down the path of good health and ask others to join you. This is not a "point the finger" message. Instead, this is a "follow me" message. Take personal responsibility for your health. Take my lead. Imitate me as I imitate Jesus.

If you're reading this, then you're already on the *PrayFit* plan. *PrayFit* is the perfect tool for you and for those you lead. Be a *PrayFit* leader. Be a *PrayFit* pastor. Lead a *PrayFit* church Body.

What will you do with the gift God has given you?

PrayFit: It Takes a Congregation

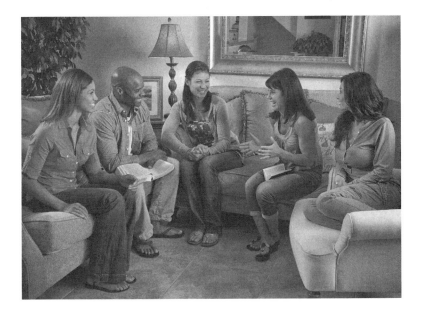

A few weeks. That is all it takes to recommit yourself to daily study in the Word and to elicit healthy change in your body. And in only minutes a day. That's the *PrayFit* challenge. Doesn't sound that daunting, does it?

Along the way, we want you both to have help and to be of help. This two-way avenue of accountability breeds measurable and marked success for those who accept the challenge, while providing a month-long, structured form of fellowship for all involved.

PrayFit can be an impactful spiritual and physical journey—one that instigates a revival of faithful, healthful living in this nation. But it takes a congregation. Here are five ways you can extend the reach of the *Pray-Fit* challenge.

1. Start a PrayFit Small Group

Grab friends, family members, fellow gym goers—anyone you think can benefit from what *PrayFit* has to offer—and go through the 28 days together. Spend dedicated time each day or each week reading, studying and praying while also logging your fitness and diet progress and encouraging each other along the way. Fitness and fellowship is a match made on earth, and one worthy of heaven.

2. Tell Your Pastor

Encourage your church leaders to bring the *PrayFit* challenge to your congregation. Charge them with setting goals for the church, such as losing a certain amount of pounds or inches, and work with the *PrayFit* team to help them meet those goals. A fitter, more faithful family is about the most God-pleasing gift we can provide Him.

3. Inspire Others

PrayFit can be something that is passed on from person to person. If it inspires you, or changes your life (or body)—and we're sure it will—and there is someone else you feel is in need of spiritual and physical transformation, then pass it on. *PrayFit* is an easy way to make a significant and lasting impression on someone's life.

4. Join the Network

Social media are a great way to help get people in the know about *PrayFit*. Set us as your home page, sign up to receive the PrayFit Daily, join us on Facebook or sign up to get the latest news at Twitter and have your friends do the same.

5. Ask Us

We're here to help. For more on how you can maximize the reach and impact of *PrayFit* within your church and community, write info@prayfit.com.

Acknowledgments

Jimmy Peña:

The Gospel Light team: Simply stated . . .
thanks for being the ones who agree.

Tina Jacobson and the B&B Media Group: You skillfully and gracefully
created partnerships, and for that, we're eternally grateful.

Erica Schultz: Thanks for superintending the entire photo shoot.
It took organization and leadership to do what we did.
Fortunately, we had you.

Michael Darter: Your masterful photography brought Prayfit.com to
life, and you did the same between these pages. Thank you, my friend.

Cindy Whitehead: Sports stylist extraordinaire. Your eye for what we wanted
and your heart for what we needed made more than you know possible.

Mike Berg: Constant editor and friend. Your timely corrections
and suggestions were invaluable.

DJ Ashba: For creating the best logo on the planet. (You really do rock.)

Thanks to the small core of devoted followers on Prayfit.com who
have been with us from the beginning. You know who you are.

Dana Angelo White: Your recipes grace our pages and will soon
change lives. Thanks for allowing us into your kitchen.

PrayFit co-authors Jimmy Page and Jim Stoppani: What can I say? You are both giants in your fields—bestselling authors, great men, and true mentors to millions . . . and to me.

Eric and Wendy Velazquez: Co-founders of PrayFit and dear friends. Your daily devotion and sacrifice will never, ever be fully regarded or rewarded this side of heaven. But I owe it to you to try.

Mario Lopez: Working with you changed my career; becoming friends with you changed my life.

Tyler Perry: The dream-giver. Without you, there's no telling; *because* of you, there's no limit.

Mom and Dad: You read what I write probably because you love me. But beyond a shadow of a doubt, I write what you read because you taught me.

My wife, Loretta: I couldn't see what God had planned 15 years ago, but I hope He plans the same for *at least* the next 50.

And to my Jesus, the one who saved my soul and made me whole. Please convince those reading this book that while life is not about the body, our health *is* a means of praise.

Jimmy Page:

Thank you to Ivelisse and our amazing kids—Jimmy, Jacob, John and Grace—for your love and support while I worked on this book.

Jim Stoppani:

I'd like to thank Jordana and my entire family for the sacrifices they made for me while working on this project.

About the Authors

Jimmy Peña, MS, received his Master's Degree in clinical exercise physiology from the University of Texas at Tyler in 1998. He then published his thesis summary on the effects of endurance training on muscle size and strength in competitive athletes in the renowned journal *Medicine & Science in Sports & Exercise*. Peña served as the fitness director for *Muscle & Fitness* and *Muscle & Fitness Hers* magazines, and for more than a decade, wrote and edited thousands of articles on training and fitness, making him one of the nation's most-published fitness experts.

In 2006, Peña designed the women's training programs for LL Cool J's *New York Times* bestseller *Platinum Workout* (Rodale Books 2006), and later that year served as creator and host of the *Muscle & Fitness* DVD series, *The Rock-Hard Challenge*. In early 2007, Peña began working with Mario Lopez, contributing to his book *Knockout Fitness* (Rodale Books 2008), while also helping prepare his physique for appearances in *People, TV Guide* and on FX's acclaimed primetime show *Nip/Tuck*. Peña is an ongoing resource for NBC's *Extra* and in 2010 was the co-author of the *New York Times* bestseller, *Extra Lean*.

Jimmy Page, MS, serves as the vice president of field ministry and national director of wellness for Fellowship of Christian Athletes. For nearly 20 years, he has been a leader in the medical fitness industry, operating wellness facilities affiliated with Sinai Hospital and Johns Hopkins. He currently hosts a daily radio segment and podcast called Fit Life Today, offering a blend of spiritual and physical health principles that promote abundant life. He's the co-author of *WisdomWalks: 40 Life-Changing Principles to Live and Give*.

Jim Stoppani, PhD, serves as senior science editor for *Muscle & Fitness*, *Muscle & Fitness Hers* and *Flex* magazines and is a science consultant for numerous companies. He has written thousands of articles on exercise, nutrition and health and is author of *The Encyclopedia of Muscle & Strength*, co-author (with LL Cool J) of *Platinum 360 Diet and Lifestyle*, and co-author of the book *Stronger Arms & Upper Body*. Dr. Stoppani is the creator of the Platinum 360 Diet and the diet program found in Mario Lopez's *Knockout Fitness*. He has been the personal nutrition and health consultant for numerous celebrity clients, including Dr. Dre, LL Cool J and Mario Lopez, and has appeared on the NBC television show *Extra* as an Extra LifeChanger.

To sign up for the PrayFit Daily, our digitally-delivered morning dose of faith and fitness, and to find additional resources for enjoying a more devoted, active lifestyle, visit us on the web at:

www.prayfit.com

To set up guest speaking appearances or to have PrayFit help you establish a fitness ministry at your church, contact us at:

PrayFit
20929 Ventura Blvd., Suite 47373
Woodland Hills, CA 91364
info@prayfit.com

Join the PrayFit Network:
Follow us at **www.twitter.com/prayfit**
Friend us at **www.facebook.com/officialprayfit**
Watch us at **www.youtube.com/prayfit**